/150

D0753603

Limit Setting in Clinical Practice

Limit Setting in Clinical Practice

Stephen A. Green, M.D. (editor)
Richard L. Goldberg, M.D.
David M. Goldstein, M.D.
Ellen Leibenluft, M.D.

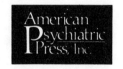

1400 K Street, N.W.
Washington, DC 20005

Copyright © 1988 American Psychiatric Press, Inc.

ALL RIGHTS RESERVED

Manufactured in the United States of America

First Edition

88 89 90 91 92 5 4 3 2 1

Library of Congress Cataloging-in-Publication Data

Limit setting in clinical practice.

Includes bibliographies.
1. Psychotherapy. 2. Psychotherapist and patient.
I. Green, Stephen A., 1945–   . [DNLM: 1. Physician-
Patient Relations. 2. Psychotherapy—methods.
WM 420 L734]
RC480.5.L55 1988   616.89'14   87-31841
ISBN 0-88048-256-7

Contents

Preface

ZETZEL'S (1968) classic paper on hysteria cautions clinicians about the therapeutic turmoil emanating from inaccurate diagnosis. She begins with a familiar nursery rhyme:

> There was a little girl
> And she had a little curl
> Right in the middle of her forehead.
> And when she was good
> She was very, very good,
> But when she was bad
> She was horrid.

This is an extremely appropriate preface to Zetzel's paper, which investigates four subtypes of "hysterics," who actually span the spectrum from neurotics with unresolved oedipal issues to individuals manifesting a borderline personality organization. Zetzel discusses the importance of correct diagnosis: It determines the direction of psychotherapy, guiding the clinician toward an introspective, anxiety-provoking approach or a more supportive stance. As suggested by the rhyme, the paper is equally concerned with *how patients behave,* inside and outside the therapeutic environment, and the effect of their actions on the treatment.

Correctly addressing patients' behaviors is an extremely important aspect of the therapeutic process. Semrad (1969) defines psychotherapy as a collaborative task that enables an individual to acknowledge, bear, and put into perspective those painful affects that adversely affect functioning and infringe upon happiness. He emphasizes the *shared responsibility* of this process: The patient must endure periods of affective distress, trusting in the judgment of a therapist who must empathically and diligently guide the patient toward progressive appreciation of unconscious conflicts and motivations. Given the mutuality of the experience, treatment will fail when a patient is more committed to acting out his feelings than to systematically investigating those emotions within the safety of a structured therapeutic environment. This conception of psychotherapy applies particularly to introspective (anxiety-provoking) work, though positive collaboration between patient and therapist is also the foundation of supportive (anxiety-suppressing) treatment. The latter relies heavily on the therapist's ability to elicit and maintain a positive transference, which is then used to educate and direct the patient and to support and enhance the patient's defensive structure (Winston et al. 1986).

Because anxiety-provoking and anxiety-suppressing psychotherapy are founded on a collaborative alliance between the participants, the impact of a patient's maladaptive behaviors can be protean—regardless of diagnostic considerations. For example, schizophrenic individuals who predominantly manifest negative symptoms of the illness may have considerable difficulties in interpersonal relationships, but may not have difficulty maintaining long-term, stable employment. On the other hand, the presence of multiple first-rank symptoms is frequently manifested in chaotic, often dangerous behaviors. Obviously, the treatment of patients from each of these groups will vary significantly, despite the fact that the affected individuals share a common disease. Within different diagnostic groups (for example, personality disorders, affective disorders, addictive disorders), a patient's responsiveness to treatment often depends on his idiosyncratic behaviors, actions influenced by myriad factors that may fluctuate constantly during the psychotherapeutic interaction.

How the clinician deals with a patient's behavior in large measure determines if treatment is a positive productive endeavor or a detrimental encounter that can precipitously or insidiously degenerate into an antitherapeutic morass. Maladaptive behaviors are first addressed via standard psychotherapeutic techniques, such as suggestion, manipulation, abreaction, clarification, and interpretation. Should these fail to stem an individual's regressive acting out, then more vigorous measures, in the form of appropriate limit setting interventions, are required. This is not to suggest that limit setting is *the* critical variable in psychotherapy. It is, however, an extremely important aspect of the complex doctor–patient interaction, and often the sole means of controlling a patient's maladaptive behaviors when they pose a threat to that patient, the therapist, or an ongoing psychotherapy. Despite this crucial role in the therapeutic process, limit setting is a relatively ill-defined subject, a situation that too often detracts from its clinical effectiveness.

The literature concerning the theoretical basis, technique, and implementation of limit setting is remarkably sparse. With few notable exceptions (Murphy and Guze 1960; Abroms 1968; Millar 1968), relevant articles are either too limited in scope (Cohen and Grinspoon 1963; Grunebaum and Klerman 1967; Graff and Mallin 1967; Adler 1973; Friedman 1975) or generally deficient. This sparseness of literature exists despite an evolution from the neutral, abstinent therapeutic stance personified by the psychoanalyst to the more active, confrontational approach of contemporary short-term therapists.

Our individual training experiences generally mirrored this inattention to limit setting. When cases began to unravel, supervisors advocated more stringent limits. A select group of teachers offered thoughtful, concrete suggestions, operationally defining an appropriate treatment approach and theoretically justifying those recommendations. More often, admonitions to set limits were devoid of any suggestions, pragmatic or otherwise, except when we were urged to use psychoactive medications and/or more stringent control by the treatment milieu when severely disorganized patients became increasingly regressed. We understood that setting appropriate limits was an intricate task; however, we felt we were being told of the need for limit setting more than we were being instructed in how to achieve that end.

Many clinicians still regard limit setting as a vague, somewhat murky process, a situation that prompted our study of the therapist's role in dealing with patients' maladaptive behaviors. Our initial interest was further sparked by recent developments in the delivery of mental health care that require the individual practitioner to be even more skilled at setting limits. Growing constraints in terms of time and financial support allotted to psychiatric treatment, as well as a decreased network of social resources, have placed greater stress on clinicians. Deinstitutionalization, decreased third party reimbursements, and the spectre of diagnosis-related groups (DRGs), require practitioners to treat all patients more quickly, regardless of how an individual's behavior may interfere with his diagnostic evaluation and/or subsequent therapy. These factors may also be implicated in the trend toward sicker patient populations: Briefer hospitalizations and abbreviated aftercare services, caused by decreases in health insurance benefits and governmental subsidies, can deprive patients of optimal treatment. These varied factors have certainly complicated the care of some individuals, particularly those whose pathology greatly impedes the psychotherapeutic process because of the maladaptive behavior it causes in them (for example, excessive withdrawal, disorganization, impulsivity, self-destructiveness) or the response to that behavior it elicits in the therapist. Clinicians are currently expected to accomplish more in less time, circumstances which highlight the value of limit setting as a fundamental therapeutic strategy.

This book was written to provide practitioners with a more comprehensive appreciation of the all-important limit setting process. Our general goal was to respond to the question, How can clinicians effectively and appropriately set limits so as to safeguard their patients, themselves, and the therapeutic process? The answer derives from investigation of several areas, which roughly parallel the chapters in this volume. Chapter 1 operationally defines the limit setting process, breaking it down into its component parts. This is presented via case material and discussion of the technical maneuvers indicated for specific maladaptive behaviors. Chapter 2 explores the theoretical underpinnings of limit setting. It identifies and organizes fundamental principles of psychodynamic and behavioral psychotherapy, illustrating how appropriate limits derive from a synthesis of these two treatment perspectives. Chapter 3 explores the transference relationship, probably the most fundamental aspect of the psychotherapeutic interaction in regard to the limit setting process. Transference and countertransference issues frequently precipitate acting out of maladaptive behaviors, and may detract from the effectiveness of standard therapeutic maneuvers used to contend with those destructive actions. The case histories illustrate how transference distortions can rapidly endanger a psychotherapy, particularly when they precipitate unhealthy countertransference responses in the therapist. Chapter 4 discusses limit setting with inpatients, a population considerably affected by the recent changes in mental health care policy. After exploring those characteristics of the treatment milieu involved in the limit setting process, the chapter discusses therapeutic strategies for common (and often dangerous) maladaptive behaviors of inpatients. Chapter 5 presents a model for teaching limit setting. It provides guidelines concerning substantive goals and addresses the process of this educational task. The import of this chapter should be particularly noted; indeed, this common deficiency of our individual training experiences was a primary stimulus for our writing this book.

We believe *Limit Setting in Clinical Practice* can benefit all mental health personnel involved in direct patient care. Psychiatric treatment is effective only when clinician and patient experience the therapeutic environment as safe and secure; consequently, it must be free of all maladaptive behaviors that could endanger either participant. This volume should provide useful theoretical and pragmatic guidelines for achieving that end in the practice of introspective and supportive psychotherapy. Our only caution is that didactic knowledge must always be supplemented with experiential learning. Patients are unique human beings, and consequently, each psychotherapy has distinctive themes, interactions, and nuances that must be appreciated and respected by the clinician. This requires case-by-case modification of limit setting interventions, a skill that cannot be learned from a book without concomitant—and considerable—practical experience.

REFERENCES

Abroms G: Setting limits. Arch Gen Psychiatry 19:113–119, 1968

Adler G: Hospital treatment of borderline patients. Am J Psychiatry 130:32–35, 1973

Cohen R, Grinspoon L: Limit setting as a corrective ego experience. Arch Gen Psychiatry 8:74–79, 1963

Friedman H: Psychotherapy of borderline patients: the influence of theory on technique. Am J Psychiatry 132:1048–1052, 1975

Graff HN, Mallin R: The syndrome of the wrist cutter. Am J Psychiatry 124:74–79, 1967

Grunebaum H, Klerman G: Wrist slashing. Am J Psychiatry 124:527–534, 1967

Millar T: Limit setting and psychological maturation. Arch Gen Psychiatry 18:214–221, 1968

Murphy M, Guze S: Setting limits: the management of the manipulative patient. Am J Psychother 14:30–47, 1960

Semrad E: A clinical formulation of the psychoses, in Teaching Psychotherapy of Psychotic Patients. Edited by Semrad E, van Buskirk D. New York, Grune and Stratton, 1969

Winston A, Pinsker H, McCullough L: A review of supportive psychotherapy. Hosp Community Psychiatry 37:1105–1114, 1986

Zetzel E: The so-called good hysteric. Int J Psychoanal 49:229–245, 1968

Chapter 1

The Art of Limit Setting

REASONED, THOUGHTFUL limit setting is a prerequisite for effective psychotherapy. In addition to being an experienced clinician, knowledgeable about various psychotherapeutic strategies and technical maneuvers, as well as the use of psychoactive medications, therapists must be skilled at imposing appropriate limits on patients, particularly when treating difficult individuals who express many of their emotions behaviorally. Though this concept is understood by most mental health personnel, the actual process of imposing limits remains vague and ill defined. As indicated in the preface, useful discussion of this topic is relatively sparse in the psychiatric literature: Some works focus on limit setting as it applies to individuals with specific diagnoses or particular clinical situations, but few offer an overview that integrates theory and practice in a comprehensive and clinically relevant fashion. As a result many therapists discover the true vagaries of this crucial aspect of psychotherapy

The decision to use the masculine pronouns throughout this book to refer in general to individuals of both sexes was seen with regret as an unavoidable requirement for readability.

1

when they treat their first seriously acting out patient. Though it has its distinctive issues, the following clinical vignette will probably evoke distressingly familiar memories:

Ms. E., a 26-year-old unmarried secretary, presented to the outpatient clinic of a university hospital complaining of severe dysphoric episodes. They began shortly after she resumed an old relationship, one which she had previously ended because of ongoing, tumultuous struggles with her boyfriend. Though she had believed he had "turned over a new leaf" the old arguments soon recurred. She begun cutting her arms with a razor when he was out of town on business and had taken a minor overdose during one of his absences. Despite a history of an intensely ambivalent symbiotic relationship with her mother and estrangement from her abusive, alcoholic father, Ms. E. had never previously sought psychiatric treatment. She was evaluated by Dr. P., a second-year resident, and judged to be "masochistic and histrionic, but not psychotic." He felt she was intelligent, verbal, and motivated to discover the cause for her dysphoria. His diagnostic impression was "dysthymic disorder in a borderline personality disorder," and he recommended twice-weekly outpatient psychotherapy. The patient was discharged to home after scheduling an appointment with Dr. P. for the following week.

While presenting the case to his supervisor, Dr. P. mentioned that Ms. E. had called him several times a day since their initial meeting. On each occasion she described different aspects of her dysphoria: She either elaborated on specific symptoms or reported suspected precipitants, such as a perceived rejection from her boyfriend or the discomfort of being alone. After offering an insightful psychodynamic formulation of the case, the supervisor admonished Dr. P. to "set strict limits" on his patient. Unfortunately, the supervisor did not specify the goals or requirements of these limits, and was somewhat vague when Dr. P. questioned him about details. The young trainee left his supervisor's office feeling frustrated and dissatisfied, worried about his ability to treat Ms. E. and generally concerned about his professional competence.

At their next meeting, Dr. P. informed his patient that she had to limit her phone calls to him. She responded by saying she felt guilty about infringing on his valuable time; however, she was terrified that the impulse to harm herself would become overwhelming and irresistible were she prohibited from calling him when she felt rejected and alone. The two of them subsequently agreed that Ms. E. could call only if she felt imminently self-destructive. Over the next few days her contact continued unabated, and the focus of her complaints shifted exclusively to self-destructive ruminations and impulses. When Dr. P. discussed this development with his supervisor, he received more detailed information concerning limit setting. He was advised to instruct Ms. E. to go to the emergency room whenever she felt self-destructive, rather than call him. Dr. P.'s directive to the patient caused her to become sullen and withdrawn during their next meeting; though she denied any negative feelings toward her therapist, by the end of the hour he felt he had failed Ms. E. by subjecting her to yet another rejection.

The patient arrived at her next session with her left wrist wrapped in gauze. When questioned about the bandage, she reluctantly reported that she had cut herself the previous evening following a fight with her boyfriend. She said that she had declined going to the emergency room because she was ashamed "to tell my story to someone who didn't know me." Dr. P. recommended immediate hospitalization, a suggestion she rejected because she "didn't want to miss work and have everyone know about my depression." She insisted that she was currently in control of herself and promised to go to the emergency room if any self-destructive impulses recurred. Later that day, Dr. P. received two phone messages from his patient stating that she felt "very suicidal." Under specific instructions from his supervisor, he called Ms. E. and insisted that she immediately admit herself to the hospital. Unlike their previous lengthy calls, Dr. P. refused to engage in any further dialogue after stating his recommendation; he told Ms. E. they would talk further after she was hospitalized. As the conversation ended he noted an obviously angry tone to her voice.

When Dr. P. arrived home several hours later, he found blood smeared on his apartment door, as well as a note from his patient saying that this was the only way she could make him comprehend the extent of her distress. Panicked, he called his supervisor, who advised enlisting the police to escort her to a hospital where she could be voluntarily or involuntarily admitted. Though Dr. P. agreed to this plan, he was haunted by a mental image of Ms. E.'s shock and betrayal when the police arrived at her door. Consequently, he called the patient directly and arranged to meet her at the emergency room, hoping he could persuade her to accept voluntary hospitalization at that time. Ms. E. was contrite and apologetic when they met; however, she adamantly rejected any suggestion that she required inpatient treatment. When Dr. P. reminded her that he had grounds to hospitalize her involuntarily, she became enraged, berating him for his insensitivity and inability "to really understand me." She asked, "How can you

possibly think about locking me up? What would that prove?" She
continued, "All it would do is make me feel more helpless and worse
about myself. If you were more experienced—if you really knew what
you were doing—you would never have suggested it. I know now that
I should never have trusted you." Having begun this meeting
determined to have his patient hospitalized, Dr. P. was now convinced
that he had permanently ruptured their working alliance. He was,
therefore, greatly relieved when Ms. E. finally made a commitment to
her safety for that night, promising to see him for an extra appointment
the following morning. The scheduled meeting never occurred. After
leaving the emergency room Ms. E. became acutely agitated, screaming
obscenities and banging her head against the walls of her apartment.
The noise prompted neighbors to call the police, who brought Ms. E.
to the hospital where she was admitted against her will. Dr. P. was
informed of these events at 4:00 A.M. when he was called by the
psychiatry resident on duty.

Some of Dr. P.'s inability to effectively set limits was due to
inexperience. Seasoned therapists generally avoid his mistakes—and
misadventures—because of their broader exposure to clinical practice. However, they are not exempt from therapeutic quagmires,
many of which occur because of errors in determining and/or
implementing appropriate limits. The crucial aspect in the management of clinicians' so-called worst cases is usually limit setting. It is
an intrinsically difficult task, made more so by inadequate didactic
training and unrecognized countertransference. Effective limit setting is an art that requires pragmatic clinical maneuvers based on a
sound theoretical foundation. Only by appreciating this blend of
the practical and theoretical can the physician achieve a knowledgeable comfort as to why, how, and when he should set limits with
patients. Before exploring the detailed stages of the limit-setting
process, the reader should first be sensitized to the general behaviors—of patients *and* therapists—that signal need for limits. They
are summarized in the following three tenets.

*The patient can either raise hell or raise his level of self-observation, but
he cannot do both simultaneously.* Every therapist has been victimized
by certain patients skilled at creating chaos in their own lives, as well
as the lives of others. Whether it is accomplished via intentional
manipulation or more unconscious mechanisms, such as splitting,
patients can effect maelstroms of struggling and fighting among

those close to them. Unfortunately, the therapist frequently becomes the clearinghouse for the pleas, accusations, threats, and ultimatums issuing from these individuals. Entanglements in situations outside the therapeutic setting, often requiring numerous and frequent contacts with family members, employers, and legal personnel, drain the therapist's energies. They also necessitate discussion of the details of these interactions with the patient; this further distracts doctor and patient from necessary psychotherapeutic work and can promote a negative countertransference characterized by feelings of frustration and distrust. Under these circumstances psychotherapy is, at best, tenuous.

The extreme difficulty in treating someone who barely talks or listens to his therapist becomes an impossibility if that individual fails to appear for scheduled appointments. Such negativistic behavior is actually a corollary of the preceding observation about limit setting, in that it is a passive means of hell-raising within the therapeutic environment. Silence, or minimal engagement in the treatment process, tests the physician's patience as much as his clinical skills. The patient's withdrawal may reflect distrust, a significant obstacle to effective treatment, but one that can usually be surmounted by an empathic, nonjudgmental approach. Withdrawal, however, can also be a more provocative communication: It may be a nonverbal challenge to the therapist to actively involve his patient in treatment despite the latter's obvious resistance. This degree of nonengagement is actually a pronouncement by the patient, his perception of the uselessness of treatment. In addition to impeding any collaborative therapeutic efforts, this stance, too, stirs an angry countertransference that may serve to further alienate the patient.

Objectivity cannot prevail in a therapeutic environment if the patient is more interested in intimidating his doctor than listening to him, and the physician feels more inclined to harm his patient than treat him. The two participants of any therapeutic relationship may knowingly or unconsciously conspire to struggle rather than to work together toward a common set of goals. Though either individual can initiate this process, it is usually precipitated by the patient's transference distortion and perpetuated by the therapist's countertransference response. The physician always bears partial responsibility for such an antitherapeutic competition; consequently, it is imperative that he recognize the contribution he makes to this vicious cycle.

Any of the above clinical situations should immediately alert the clinician to the need for effective limit setting. Webster's dictionary defines limits as "boundaries" that "terminate, circumscribe, or confine," an accurate representation of their role in psychotherapy. Limits draw territorial lines between the patient and therapist, the patient and significant people in his life, and the very special nature of the psychotherapeutic setting and the everyday world. These are not vague, amorphous boundaries easily subject to change. Rather, they are explicitly stated guidelines that define appropriate interactions of the patient and enunciate the realistic expectations of treatment. Limit setting becomes necessary when a patient's maladaptive behavior poses a threat to someone, usually himself and/or his therapist, or when it jeopardizes the ongoing psychotherapeutic process (Murphy and Guze 1960). The physician's first response to such situations is intervention via standard clinical maneuvers, such as clarification or interpretation (Bibring 1954). Unfortunately, these measures are often inadequate because the patient's acting out behavior is too gratifying; the relief it provides from emotional tension is often a disincentive to pursue the sometimes painful work of psychotherapy (Graff and Mallin 1967). This in turn can heighten the therapist's countertransference and feelings of anxiety, inadequacy, frustration, and hopelessness, which may further underline the therapeutic alliance (Goldberg 1983). The only resolution to such a therapeutic impasse is consistent implementation of carefully drawn boundaries.

The general schema for setting limits involves the following steps. First, the therapist points out the maladaptive behavior that is threatening the psychotherapy, the patient, or the therapist himself. Next, the therapist delineates the precise limits to which he believes treatment can withstand that behavior. Finally, he specifically defines the consequences of the patient's continued actions (Murphy and Guze 1960). The central element of this process is the formation of an alliance between the therapist's ego and the healthier aspect of the patient's ego. As the following clinical vignette illustrates, this permits the adult-to-adult interaction necessary for productive work in psychotherapy.

> Mr. B., a middle-aged businessman, appeared for a psychiatric consultation with a thick casing of mud encrusted on his shoes. As he

related a history of always feeling victimized by others, he ground his soiled shoes into the physician's carpet, producing a large dirt stain. Angered by the man's actions and judging that he had exceeded the bounds of acceptable behavior, the therapist warned Mr. B. against further soiling his carpet. This admonition had only a transitory effect, and consequently, the therapist subsequently informed his patient that he would have to leave the office if he did not remove his shoes or curtail the spread of mud. Startled by such candor, Mr. B. slowly began to untie his shoelaces while simultaneously complaining about the physician's excessive fastidiousness. The therapist replied that if what he had just witnessed was representative of the patient's usual behavior, he could easily imagine such insensitivity triggering criticism and/or rejection from others in his life. He wondered if that type of interpersonal pattern might contribute to the patient's sense of persecution. After initially rejecting the hypothesis as ludicrous, Mr. B. began to reflect on in, ultimately resulting in a productive session.

This vignette illustrates several important issues concerning the *why* of limit setting, the theoretical basis for imposing therapeutic boundaries that is explored in detail in Chapter 2. First, by informing Mr. B. that he considered his office an important extension of himself, the therapist communicated his sense of self-worth. This trait, necessary to successfully persevere in any endeavor, is particularly relevant to the therapeutic relationship, which is destined to disintegrate if a patient does not respect his physician. Second, by placing a boundary on Mr. B.'s objectionable behavior, the therapist indicated his intolerance of all circumstances that interfere with his ability to function optimally. This communicated a dedication to his work and, by implication, the seriousness he attached to his patients' complaints. Third, by linking Mr. B.'s behavior in the office with potential consequences in his daily life, the therapist underscored his intention not to ignore behaviors which he judged to be obviously detrimental to the businessman's overall interpersonal relationships. Moreover, this informed the patient that such difficulties could be examined, and ultimately understood, within a therapeutic environment made safe by the imposition of appropriate limits—an appealing alternative to the self-defeating struggles he provoked in retaliation for perceived rejections. Finally, by imposing limits on a behavior which he experienced as personally insulting and, consequently, an impediment to treatment, the therapist declared his intention to act similarly when *any* of the patient's behaviors impacted negatively on their collaborative work. This put his patient on notice that he was expected to consistently stick to the therapeutic task. In addition, it offered him the reassurance that his doctor would be vigilant and respond with action if he felt the patient's emotions might evolve into behaviors detrimental to either of them.

The fundamental principle behind the *how* of limit setting is clear identification of the specific maladaptive behaviors that need to be altered and equally precise articulation of the consequences if those behaviors persist. Maladaptive actions fall into the general categories of withdrawn, disorganized, destructive, and unwise or demanding and manipulative behavior. In any of these circumstances, the clinician must clearly delineate the impediment to the collaborative work between doctor and patient, and then state the limits to which the psychotherapy can tolerate that behavior. Ideally, therapeutic boundaries should be few in number. When several behaviors are simultaneously targeted, it becomes more difficult for a single practitioner or ward staff to implement those limits consistently and, consequently, harder for individuals to adhere to them. In addition, patients frequently feel victimized by excessive limits. Experiencing such limits as punishment, an overpowering assault, patients are less likely to respond therapeutically. If more than one behavior requires limits, the therapist ideally should prioritize instead of imposing numerous injunctions simultaneously.

In order to ensure clarity, limits also need to be restated to patients, as well as to adjunctive staff. This is a prophylactic intervention designed to prevent the recurrences of maladaptive behaviors that frequently return after a period of quiescence. The therapist should periodically reaffirm the treatment contract by reminding all concerned of the specific acting out that has been targeted for specific consequences. Reiteration, however, should not be too frequent. Repetitive injunctions against particular activities often become self-defeating; the patient may feel more provoked than reassured, or doubtful as to his therapist's conviction to implement designated limits.

If the therapist lacks clarity in his thinking or communications to individuals concerning behaviors that must be curtailed, his interventions may actually confuse and disorganize patients rather than facilitate the psychotherapy. The negative impact of such poorly imposed limits is evident in the initial phase of the following case:

Mrs. C., a 25-year-old woman with a severe borderline personality organization, had reverted to carving wounds into her forearms with knives and razor blades during a period of enhanced stress. Her therapist attempted to control this behavior via interpretation addressing its meaning via-à-vis their relationship, as well as to a recent separation in her life. When this intervention failed, he informed Mrs. C. that he viewed her self-inflicted mutilations as a potential threat to her survival and essentially ordered her to abandon the behavior regardless of any degree of tension she was experiencing. His action, motivated in large measure by unrecognized countertransference feelings of helplessness and frustration, was also ineffective.

The therapist eventually informed Mrs. C. that her actions threatened the continuation of treatment. He declared that he would require the patient to show him her forearms at the start of each therapy session and that if he observed evidence of one more wound he would insist on immediate hospitalization. Further, he would not meet with her while hospitalized, nor would he continue as her physician if she refused hospitalization under the guidelines he had just set out. The patient discontinued this self-destructive behavior after hearing her therapist's explicit limits and the consequences of continued misbehavior. She then began a long period of angry denunciaion of her physician, declaring that she had felt increasingly rejected by him as he commended her on her steady progress toward more independent functioning. Though her response was difficult for the therapist to bear, it proved a fruitful focus of treatment and enabled the psychotherapeutic process to proceed.

Despite the clarity with which limits are imposed, individuals may still ascribe broader meaning to a therapist's interventions. For example, when a young male patient was told that the incessant phone calls to his female therapist had to stop, he angrily condemned her as cold and uncaring. Another patient might be made anxious by such a limit, viewing it as an attempt to curtail his overall autonomy, whereas yet another could respond with the depression characteristic of narcissistic injury and deflated self-esteem (Abroms 1968). For this reason, it is important that limit setting engage what practitioners of transactional analysis would define as the "adult part of" the patient. In this ego state, the patient is more capable of observing the manifestations and consequences of his maladaptive behavior; such understanding is the first step toward gaining control over it. Conversely, when limits are made to sound like parental injunctions, the converse pattern—the dependent child—is reinforced in the patient. Thus, when setting limits, the therapist must always speak to the healthier, adult side of his patient, in order to enhance observing ego. The following vignette illustrates the positive effects of setting limits in a manner that augments the patient's higher level of ego functioning, in this instance by actively involving him in the limit setting process.

> Mr. S., a 28-year-old architect with a borderline personality disorder, was hospitalized with depression precipitated by impending legal action for assaulting a patron in a bar. Two previous hospitalizations were required when episodes of binge drinking resulted in his considerable loss of impulse control. During each inpatient stay, he had gone to a bar while on pass and had returned to the ward inebriated and argumentative. Mr. S.'s therapist confronted the patient with his alcohol abuse, explicitly emphasizing his repetitive drinking pattern while in the hospital. After mutually agreeing that alcohol was largely responsible for most of Mr. S.'s problems, his therapist asked him to think about what consequences should ensue if he were to again abuse alcohol while hospitalized. Mr. S. and his therapist eventually concurred that the first infraction would result in the loss of all inpatient privileges for a week, and that the next infraction would result in immediate administrative discharge. Predictably, the patient returned inebriated from an evening pass, and he was immediately restricted to the ward for one week. Rather than responding as he had in the past, like a petulant, accusing child who felt unfairly treated by an authoritarian parent, Mr. S. was able to reflect on the earlier collaboraton with his therapist in determining the appropriate response for continued drinking. He became noticeably depressed, increasingly critical of his self-destructive potential, and gravely concerned about his future given the real possibility of a prison sentence for his last drunken assault. There were no other incidents concerning his use of alcohol during the remainder of his hospital stay.

Providing a patient with the opportunity to share some responsibility when establishing limits can help mobilize higher level adaptive and defensive mechanisms. This fosters a greater sense of control over his affects and impulses, positively influences current behavior vis-à-vis the psychotherapy, and instructs the patient as to similar compromises and negotiations he must effect with people in his everyday life. The effectiveness of limit setting depends heavily on the *when* of a therapist's interventions. If limits are imposed too quickly, the clinician is often perceived as the fulfillment of the patient's worst introject, namely, the primitive, withdrawing object. Conversely, delayed or infrequent limits often promote serious regression, with its consequent effects on the patient's well-being. The timing of limit setting is a complex determination affected by issues endemic to the patient (for example, his psychopathology, basic personality structure, and the extent of his maladaptive behavior), the therapist (for example, countertransference issues), and the interplay between the two of them.

The seriousness of a patient's acting out behavior is one important factor affecting what time in the treatment therapeutic boundaries are established. Ominous self-destructive acts or rigid resistances that threaten the viability of the psychotherapeutic contract obviously require immediate attention by the therapist. In general, he decides when to impose boundaries on a particular behavior by drawing on his didactic understanding of the patient and his clinical instincts—though the timing of these interventions may sometimes be affected by broader issues of the treatment. The presence of a positive working alliance, for example, greatly enhances the possibility that the therapist's interventions will result in the desired outcome. This is because the setting of any limits carries a core communication from the physician that the therapeutic relationship is in jeopardy. If a patient values his treatment he will be more inclined to abandon behavior targeted as maladaptive. The phase a psychotherapy is in also has bearing on this. At its inception the patient is relatively unfamiliar with his therapist and has little data with which to evaluate the treatment process. As a result, he may be less inclined to adhere to any directives from the physician, as illustrated in the following clinical vignette.

Ms. R., a 29-year-old divorced woman, was seen in consultation because "my life is coming apart again." She lived a chaotic existence and had several times begun treatment with a number of therapists, which she said she terminated when "things began to look brighter." In fact, in each instance she had made outlandishly excessive demands upon her physicians that culminated in a variety of temper tantrums when she did not get her way. The postscript to each of her explosions was a unilateral decision to terminate treatment. After obtaining this history, her current psychiatrist told Ms. R. that he would inform her if he felt she were making excessive demands on him so that together they could examine her behavior. Furthermore, he would terminate therapy if she acted as she had with a previous therapist when she had felt neglected, that is, refusing to leave his office until the police were called. Though sullen and sulking, the patient indicated that she would comply with these limits. However, she failed to appear for a follow-up appointment and ignored efforts to contact her.

Another aspect of treatment that affects the timing of limit setting is the psychotherapeutic work done preparatory to establishing those limits. Whenever feasible, confrontive and interpretive interventions should precede the imposition of limits, since these maneuvers afford the patient greater flexibility in exercising his own autonomy and discretion. When unacceptable behaviors are identified, the patient may modify those actions absent any injunctions from his therapist, thereby acquiring an opportunity for mastery and enhanced self-esteem. This also minimizes the potential for a dependent regression that may accompany the imposition of external controls, a more likely occurrence if limits appear disconnected from the current psychotherapeutic work. In that situation, the patient often interprets such directives as an indication of his impaired ability to function independently. Limits preceding interpretations may be incorrectly perceived as pronouncements of suboptimal functioning, particularly with a psychologically healthier patient, which can foster an inaccurate assessment of his own capacities.

The timing of limit setting is considerably influenced by countertransference issues (Grunebaum and Klerman 1967). Some clinical situations incite such frustration, anxiety, resentment, or hopelessness in the physician that he becomes unwilling, consciously or unconsciously, to permit further increments in the therapeutic tension. He may thereby curtail useful clinical interaction and/or enhance the patient's sense of perceived helplessness, by imposing therapeutic boundaries too rapidly. The potential for such occurrences is considerable, given the fact that many limits are set during a state of emotional turmoil for the therapist.

The opposite side of the countertransference issue can also affect the timing of limit setting interventions. Psychologic issues idiosyncratic to the clinician may impede the appropriate response to patients' maladaptive behaviors. This is evident in the following vignette, which illustrates the antitherapeutic effects of a clinician's reaction formation to his own assertiveness.

> Mr. P. was a 45-year-old depressed man whose excessive dependency was reflected in numerous phone calls to his therapist throughout the week. Rationalizing the necessity of "meeting the patient where he is," the therapist tolerated this behavior for some time. He considered it the necessary price for engaging the patient in a productive working alliance. As the calls became more frequent the physician's irritation also increased, accompanied by a sense of guilt for the degree of anger he held toward Mr. P. He did not set the indicated limits, but rather explained to himself that he needed a clearer psychodynamic understanding of his patient's behavior before verbalizing his own anger. To impose boundaries at this point, he reasoned, would be to act out his aggression toward the patient. His patient's continued inappropriate behavior eventually forced the therapist to act.

A thorough understanding of the component parts of limit setting—the why, how, and when of this necessary therapeutic process—is essential if the therapist expects to help patients contain or eradicate maladaptive, self-defeating behaviors. By correctly defining and imposing therapeutic boundaries, the clinician provides the patient with a dyadic model different from past object relationships, one in which the therapist is seen as neither omnipotent nor helpless in the face of intense, often threatening drives. He neither engulfs nor abandons his patient, but rather helps that individual define a new set of selective identifications that ultimately strengthens his capacity to delay, anticipate, and tolerate powerful, distressing affects. This promotes ego development (for example, reality testing and the capacity to differentiate self from others) and, consequently, more responsible, autonomous functioning.

REFERENCES

Abroms G: Setting limits. Arch Gen Psychiatry 19:113–119, 1968

Bibring E: Psychoanalysis and the dynamic psychotherapies. J Am Psychoanal Assoc 2:745–770, 1954

Cohen R, Grinspoon L: Limit setting as a corrective emotional experience. Arch Gen Psychiatry 8:90–95, 1963

Goldberg R: Psychodynamics of limit setting with the borderline patient. Am J Psychoanal 48:71–75, 1983

Graff H, Mallin R: The syndrome of the wrist cutter. Am J Psychiatry 124:74–79, 1967

Grunebaum H, Klerman G: Wrist slashing. Am J Psychiatry 124:113– 120, 1967

Murphy G, Guze S: Setting limits: the management of the manipulative patient. Am J Psychother 14:30–47, 1960

Millar T: Limit setting and psychological maturation. Arch Gen Psychiatry 18:214–221, 1968

Wolfe N: Setting reasonable limits on behavior. Am J Nursing 37:104–106, 1960

Chapter 2
The Theory of Limit Setting

*I*N HIS STUDY of the psychotherapeutic process, Jerome Frank (1961) discusses varied belief systems that facilitate and legitimize the interaction of caretakers and those seeking assistance. He demonstrates the importance of a clear rationale for the exchange between patients and clinicians, indicating how treatment suffers when that theoretical underpinning is lacking. The purpose of this chapter is to provide that necessary conceptual framework for the limit-setting process. It derives from two overlapping treatment perspectives, the psychodynamic and the behavioral approaches. The interplay between technical interventions from each of these therapeutic strategies constitutes the mechanism for change when limits are imposed during a psychotherapy.

THE PSYCHODYNAMIC PERSPECTIVE

Individuals who repeatedly require limit setting in order to remain in a psychotherapeutic relationship, and to function effectively in their daily lives, usually occupy the most disturbed segment of the diagnostic spectrum. As Kernberg (1970) notes, these so-called difficult patients suffer from significant character pathology (for example, borderline personality organization) or frank psychotic disorders. The psychodynamic orientation considers identity diffusion, or loss of a sense of self, as their overriding concern.

Because of poor differentiation between self and non-self, the fear of loss of self is reflected in a fear of the loss of external objects. (This is in contrast to healthier patients in whom the predominant issues concern competition, guilt, shame, and retaliatory punishment.) Many subsequent maladaptive behaviors are understood to be a manifestation of the accompanying anxiety (Erickson 1956; Kernberg 1970; Frosch 1970). Thus, a major goal of limit setting is reinforcement of the patient's sense of self.

The predominant psychic mechanism that protects against pathologic identity diffusion is the ability to experience *libidinal object constancy*. This metapsychological construct refers to one's capacity to maintain interpersonal relationships in the face of frustrated wishes and needs, which requires an individual to perceive himself and others as "whole objects" with an integration of both "good" and "bad" attributes. Healthier individuals have the ability to readily tolerate ambivalence and thus are able to comfortably experience themselves as autonomous beings who do not require the security of supposed "all-good" nurturers, nor protection from presumed "all-bad" persecutors. Less healthy patients, who are handicapped in their ability to maintain stable libidinal attachments, are more inclined to view the world in the extremes of unqualified good or bad.

Libidinal object constancy is theoretically achieved during the separation-individuation stage of development (Mahler 1971). Developmental impasses, which may result from infantile trauma (for example, loss of a parent or prolonged illness), mismatching between the caretaking capacity of parents and the needs of the infant (Goldberg et al. 1985), or genetic factors, interfere with this psychological maturation and predispose an individual to experience all separations as the *destruction* of a relationship. As adults, these individuals experience intensely uncomfortable affects when stressed by the loss of a love object. Their subsequent regression of psychological organization often precipitates seriously maladaptive behaviors that span the spectrum from dangerous acting out to frank psychosis. The severity of these behaviors depends in large measure on the patient's capacity for reality testing. This fundamental ego function permits one to separate one's personal contribution to a perception from external stimuli; in other words, it permits clear differentiation of self and non-self. Stress-related disruptions of reality testing are often reversible in lower level character types, such as Frosch's (1970) "psychotic character" or Kernberg's (1970) "borderline personality." The regression to psychosis can often be reversed via limit setting interventions that target characteristic ego mechanisms that distort the assessment of reality, such as splitting and projective identification. Therapeutic boundaries that specifically address these lower level mechanisms help the individual regain his capacity to accurately moderate between the realities of everyday life and the primitive impulses brought on by a feared loss of self.

Splitting describes an individual's tendency to dichotomize mental activities—affects, cognitions, and memories—into extremes of black or white. It applies to internalized object representations, as well as to intellectual precepts, such as political beliefs. Splitting functions by preserving the relationship with "good objects" at the expense of the relationship with "bad objects." Emotional contact with external objects, as well as with the self, is maintained by disavowing all negative feelings and attributing them elsewhere. In the extreme, this produces a psychosis that requires psychotherapeutic and/or pharmacologic interventions. However, splitting is present in many characterologically impaired individuals who rely on absolutist thinking to function on a nonpsychotic level and prevent disintegration of the sense of self. *Projective identification* often serves the same function in this group of patients. This complex ego mechanism first requires denial of an unacceptable wish. The individual then projects the impulse onto someone in his close environment, and finally acts in a fashion that elicits a response from the other person which validates the original projection. Inherent in this process is a blurring of the boundaries between the two individuals, which is a regressive step toward dedifferentiation. As with splitting, this process often represents a desperate effort to prevent the loss of emotional connectedness with the love object and the self. The following case illustrates how appropriate limit setting can be implemented to neutralize the maladaptive consequences of these primitive ego mechanisms.

Mrs. W., a 35-year-old married woman, began treatment because of a phobia that prevented her from getting on an airplane to travel to a family reunion. She was afraid that once in the air the plane would explode and crash, and she and her husband would die a terrifying, painful death. The trip had been arranged to celebrate her father's 65th birthday, and there was considerable pressure on Mrs. W. and her siblings to attend the party.

During the intake interview, Mrs. W. was completely unaware of the reasons for the onset of her "overwhelming fear of flying." As therapy progressed, however, it became increasingly obvious that the patient maintained a highly ambivalent assessment of herself, which was reflected in her equally polarized view of most of her interpersonal relationships. She perceived her father as sadistically controlling, particularly cold and demeaning toward women. She denied any tenderness toward him, dismissed his considerable accomplishments, and negated any of his attempts to bridge the distance between them. For example, she interpreted his many gifts exclusively as attempts to extend power and dominance over his children. Whereas Mrs. W. frequently reported that she hated her father, she saw her mother as an all-loving figure deserving of continuous praise. Any shortcomings were explained away by the patient as reactions to the tyranny of her husband. This tendency toward splitting extended to Mrs. W.'s view of herself, causing her difficulty integrating her various roles of mother, career woman, daughter, and wife. She would alternately loathe herself for various shortcomings or bask in a breezy self-acceptance, puzzled at her periods of self-criticism. Predictably, she incorporated her therapist into the black-and-white matrix. Mrs. W. immediately idealized the therapeutic relationship, denying any negative feelings toward her doctor. When this was pointed out to her, she used considerable intellectualization and reaction formation to inhibit the expression of even mild irritation.

Several months into treatment, the therapist noticed the patient's apparent weight loss. When he inquired about it, Mrs. W. reported that she had intentionally shed 20 pounds since she began treatment. She had initiated a highly ritualized diet in an attempt to correct what sounded like a severely distorted body image. Moreover, she completely denied the possibility that her actions posed any hazard to her health. The therapist had little success when he attempted to explore and understand the meaning of his patient's continuing anorexia, which he assumed represented the acting out of feelings generated by the psychotherapy. Consequently, when Mrs. W.'s weight fell to 90 pounds he decided that a limit had to be set on her self-destructive behavior. The therapist informed Mrs. W. that he would terminate the treatment unless she agreed to a comprehensive medical evaluation (which she had avoided until then) and regular follow-up visits, and allowed him to freely communicate with her internist. In addition, if her weight continued to decline, or if she developed any significant medical sequelae from her condition, she would have to accept hospitalization. After considerable protest, the patient agreed to these therapeutic boundaries, and eventually involved herself actively in the collaborative work of therapy.

During subsequent months the dynamics of Mrs. W.'s anorexia were investigated. Early in the treatment she had attempted to get the therapist to rescue her in a decisive way that would demonstrate his care and concern. However, whenever he was drawn into this type of interaction she repudiated his efforts. For example, she became depressed and withdrawn when he recommended that she be evaluated medically for her weight loss. The patient had recreated with the therapist her usual interaction with her father. Projective identification enabled her to make the therapist act like a caring father, behavior she found so threatening that she progressively withdrew from treatment via her preoccupation with dietary rituals. Mrs. W. denied herself gratification of the wish to be cared for by the father/therapist because recognition of that impulse was so antithetical to the prevailing relationships with her parents that it posed a threat of loss of her sense of self. Her anorexia was both an expression of her repudiated wish to be loved by her father and an effort to control the emergence of that wish into awareness. Her excessive weight loss was actually a maladaptive behavioral attempt to maintain the ego splitting that prevailed in her self and object relationships.

Limit setting with Mrs. W. required the therapist to "lend" her some of his own judgment, as well as to establish strict boundaries within which her markedly divergent feelings could exist. By limiting further acting out of her conflict, this combination ultimately helped her recognize troublesome unconscious issues within the safety of a controlled setting. Her capacity for self-observation—and consequently, her self/non-self differentiation—was greatly enhanced because her drive toward indiscriminate action was blocked.

Other aspects of impaired ego functioning that respond to therapeutic boundaries are the patient's capacity to assess internal and external reality and the ability to control feelings that are generated by those perceptions. The *sense of reality* refers to how one perceives oneself within one's environment. An individual may feel that he is unreal (depersonalization) or that the world around him is unreal (derealization). Persistence of this ego disturbance suggests the presence of a psychotic diagnosis; however, transient disturbances are common in patients with severe character pathology who are additionally stressed by such diverse factors as drug and alcohol use or the lack of sufficient structure in their daily lives.

One's *relationship to reality* concerns the ability to perceive what is happening internally versus externally, as opposed to testing the validity of the perception. For example, a distorted relationship to reality might cause an individual to respond to a hallucination or believe a delusional thought. Disturbances in an individual's sense of reality and relationship to reality reflect regression to an undifferentiated state where the boundary between self and non-self becomes blurred in the mind of the individual. Limit setting helps identify and reestablish that tenuous boundary.

Impulse control, the capacity to delay gratification of a wish by interposing thought and judgment between the impulse and an action, is often compromised in patients who struggle to maintain libidinal object constancy. When stressed by the fear of loss of self, these individuals frequently express their intense anxiety via destructive and generally unwise behaviors. Impulse control is actually a function of various aspects of the psychic apparatus, including autonomous ego functions (such as memory, motility, and perception) and superego activity. In regard to the latter, the prohibitions and ideals internalized by an individual at the time of resolution of the oedipal phase can either help or hinder his ability to neutralize sexual and aggressive drives (Hartmann et al. 1946; Hartmann 1962). There may also be a constitutional component that contributes to the intensity of expression of impulses (Kernberg 1970). Limit setting plays several roles in regard to impaired impulse control. First, by helping to enhance the patient's observing ego it highlights the maladaptive aspects of impulsive actions while simultaneously identifying more acceptable and productive behavioral responses to stress. It also exposes the patient to a firm, but nonpunitive, authority figure in the person of the therapist, who can be internalized as an alternative to less healthy parental models that served as the basis for superego development.

The following case history illustrates how the combination of excessive stress and specific ego deficits contributed to the patient's

failure to maintain his sense of self. As the clinical material illustrates, therapeutic boundaries specifically addressed his impaired
ability to assess reality.

Mr. J., a 25-year-old single male, began treatment after a brief
hospitalization for a transient psychotic episode. The patient had joined
a private security force soon after graduating from high school. During
a two-week course of training, conducted on the grounds of a military
facility located several hundred miles from his home, he became
progressively isolated from his peers and increasingly suspicious of
their motives. He began to worry that his fellow cadets were gaining
control over him in order to force him into performing some unnamed
act. His tension built to a fever pitch until he panicked and jumped
through a dormitory window in an effort to flee his presumed
persecutors. Mr. J. was apprehended by the local authorities and briefly
hospitalized at a nearby psychiatric facility. He recovered rapidly, but
because some of his fears persisted he began individual psychotherapy
when he returned home.

During the course of treatment, the dynamics of Mr. J.'s impulsive
acting out became increasingly clear. The middle child in a family
where academic achievement was highly prized, he was always a slow
student because of a learning disability that was not diagnosed until he
was in junior high school. This handicap, coupled with prominent
characterologic traits of passivity and dependency, greatly interfered
with his intellectual development and ultimate scholastic success. He
was limited in the ability to delay gratification, plan for the future,
reason abstractly, exercise judgment, and remember information. These
deficits periodically interfered with his capacity to test reality, in that
his thinking had a characteristic black-and-white, all-or-nothing quality
to it.

During his training experience, Mr. J.'s impaired reality testing
combined with other ego deficits in a manner that severely limited his
ability to contain his frightening impulses. He projected onto the peer
group the wish to be supported and urged into participating in the
training exercise, which served as a counterweight to his own passivity.
However, he was unable to cognitively validate this external
perception and rationally subject it to other available information
concerning the training experience. As a result, he could not effectively
delay the impulses that accompanied his misperceptions, namely, to flee
what he imagined was excessive control by his peers. Lacking healthier
ego mechanisms, such as repression, rationalization, and sublimation,
he could only see his stress-filled world in all-or-nothing terms and

converted his fear into the action of jumping through the dormitory window.

The need for limit setting with Mr. J. became apparent soon after treatment began. Despite compliant participation in the therapy, he was late in paying his first three bills. Exploration of the behavior was unproductive until the therapist threatened to terminate his services unless he received timely payment. Further discussion revealed the patient's limited ability to control his finances or negotiate the process of insurance reimbursement. He spent money on whims, and though he had no savings he genuinely believed that he would never be held accountable for his debts. This lack of thought between impulse and action paralleled his behavior at the training camp. Limit setting initially focused on the identification of specific ego deficits concerned with memory, calculation, organization, planning, and judgment. It highlighted his difficulty appreciating the consequences of spending and in addition addressed associated superego deficits that derived from an identification with his father. The therapist also attempted to minimize the development of transference distortions, given Mr. J.'s impaired ability to test reality and his subsequent potential for an unworkable psychotic transference reaction. To achieve this particular boundary, the clinician maintained a high level of activity with the patient, regularly articulated reality factors in the therapeutic relationship, and actively involved the family in the treatment. His interactive approach was designed to maintain a dissonance between projection and reality sufficient to contain the patient's regression to psychosis.

Heinz Kohut (1971, 1972) discusses a final area of deficient ego functioning that requires active limit setting in order to help individuals maintain a stable sense of self. His study of narcissism identified an intrapsychic structure that he termed the *grandiose self,* an infantile construct central to the regulation of self-esteem. The grandiose self, which has a boundless need to be admired and praised, feels depressed and worthless when its wishes are frustrated. Disappointments caused by the unrealistic desire for limitless power often leads to inner- or outer-directed explosions of narcissistic rage. This usually takes the form of impulsive acting out in difficult patients, who experience any degree of diminished self-esteem as a devastating narcissistic injury. The acting out frequently has an expansive, omnipotent quality, which may serve to compensate for the injured self-esteem (Berkowitz 1977). An individual's pathologic grandiosity, which is actually a form of reality distortion, persists during a psychotherapy until challenged by clearly stated therapeutic boundaries that prepare the way for the development of enhanced observing ego (Kernberg 1967, 1970). The following case is an example of such an encounter.

Dr. Y., a 40-year-old scientist, began treatment because of recurrent depressions, failure to sustain a heterosexual relationship, and periods of work inhibition. His self-esteem was largely dependent on the recognition and praise he was able to generate from the people in his life, as well as his association with several prestigious institutions and individuals in positions of power. This pattern was soon established in the treatment, which quickly became a stage for humorously recounting his life's misadventures instead of seriously focusing on his emotional distress. The therapist was initially seduced by the patient's manner. He found himself laughing at Dr. Y.'s self-mockery and enjoying reports of his entangled sexual escapades. It was not until the patient began frequent business trips out of the city that the therapist responded appropriately to his patient's maladaptive behaviors. He recognized that therapy had degenerated to a series of sporadic meetings that sounded more like travelogues, since Dr. Y. always returned with some amusing story that he would insist on reporting during much of the session.

At this point, the therapist recognized the need for explicit limits that he outlined to his patient with an explanation of why they were necessary. He would continue the treatment only if Dr. Y. arranged his business schedule so that it did not interfere with therapy sessions. Dr. Y.'s response was a temper tantrum, during which he accused the therapist of wanting to end their relationship because he really found him boring. This began a period when the two of them jointly explored the patient's excessive need to be admired, respected, and loved. His acting out behaviors, which were in response to projected feelings of indifference or criticism by the therapist, had a grandiose quality designed to impress the clinician. However, this romanticized vision of himself caused him repeated disappointment and unhappiness in his daily life and now threatened the psychotherapy. His distorted sense of reality about himself, aggravated by some difficulties in impulse control, made interpretive work untenable without the additional support of therapeutic boundaries that addressed his various ego deficits. Dr. Y.'s subsequent success in maintaining a stable libidinal attachment to the therapist resulted in considerable clinical progress.

To varying degrees, all patients look to the therapist to offset disappointment, satisfy interpersonal needs, and provide what has been lacking in object relationships. Many patients come to recognize, and eventually control, what they contribute to their unhappiness. Others are not as discerning. Weakened ego functioning causes so-called difficult patients to rapidly ascribe clinicians the role of omniscient, powerful providers. Rather then viewing the therapist as a separate individual with professional responsibilities that are distinct from his own wishes and needs, this type of patient perceives the clinician as his exclusive mainstay of support and succor—a stance reflecting poor self/non-self differentiation. When the clinician meets the patient's demands, or is perceived in fantasy as fulfilling desired hopes, he is regarded as the "all good" provider, and the patient is then content and clinically stable. When the clinician is viewed as distant and authoritarian, often occurring during actual separations or periods of perceived rejections, the patient becomes intensely anxious and acts out accordingly. His exaggerated reactivity, making him alternately devouring and repelling, places the clinician in an extremely precarious position. The psychotherapy will not survive without appropriate limits based on a comprehensive appreciation of the patient's various ego deficits.

THE BEHAVIORAL PERSPECTIVE

According to Skinner (1953), learning can be defined as "a change in the probability of response" that occurs when one specifies the conditions under which altered behavior comes about. Though his theory derived from laboratory research concerned with objective observable facts about the learning process, it validates a model of behavioral psychotherapy that is particularly useful when dealing with patients whose treatment requires explicit limits. Individuals who resort to maladaptive behaviors rely heavily on preverbal methods to alleviate anxiety, and consequently, a successful treatment must also include *action* on the part of the clinician. The behavioral interventions derived from learning theory can provide that essential factor, via such techniques as reinforcement, conditioning, modeling, and shaping.

The central tenets of learning theory rest on the observations of the well-known Russian physiologist, Ivan Pavlov, who identified what is now accepted as classical conditioning. In his laboratory setting, an unconditioned stimulus (meat) produced an unconditioned response (salivation) in dogs. Pavlov elicited a conditioned response (salivation) when the arrival of the meat was paired with a conditioned stimulus (the ringing of a bell). Moreover, that conditioning could be ablated via the phenomenon of extinction when the meat was repeatedly withheld after ringing the bell.

Pavlov's observations became the basis of operant conditioning, in which varied stimuli evoke behavioral responses that are not automatic. In this process, an organism learns to perform a specific task in order to receive a reward. For example, a pigeon may learn to press a bar to receive food, or a patient may learn to threaten suicide in order to capture the attention of his therapist. The continuation of such behavior is determined by the nature of reinforcement. Positive reinforcement refers to a response that increases the likelihood of the recurrence of a specific event, whereas negative reinforcement refers to an opposite response. Further refinement of operant conditioning has led to the clinically pragmatic concept of shaping, in which behavior is altered in a stepwise fashion. The therapist identifies a desired outcome, designates the steps necessary to achieve that goal, and guides the individual's behavior in the desired direction via sequencing of conditioning. Progress is similarly rewarded in a stepwise fashion. The technique allows patients to learn new behaviors incrementally rather than requiring them to dramatically effect such changes.

A final behavioral phenomenon that has widespread clinical applicability is modeling. This is a form of learning by imitation that can affect cognitive processes, emotional expression, and specific actions. Modeling can be used to foster healthy responses to problem situations and/or limit self-defeating behaviors. In modeling, an "effect of the person" enhances one's learning. This concept, similar to the dynamic concept of transference, is a recognition that the feeling a subject has toward the model can affect the learning that takes place. For example, an individual can develop more appropriate means of discharging aggressive impulses by observing the reactions of a therapist whom he admires.

Learning theory is involved in the limit setting process in several ways. First, therapeutic boundaries delineate unacceptable behaviors to patients and then serve to inhibit and extinguish those patterned maladaptive responses. In addition to preserving the psychotherapy, this provides an opportunity for healthier behaviors to emerge. Second, positive reinforcement is often necessary if these newer, more adaptive behaviors are to persist. This usually requires the clinician's verbal support, such as praise for a patient who declares feelings of rejection openly as opposed to his previous method of communicating the affect, self-mutilatory behavior. Therapists also effect positive reinforcement by bestowing privileges or compliments. This behavioral intervention fosters clinical progression and decreases the incidence of acting out in the present and future, as illustrated by the following vignette:

> Ms. K., a 40-year-old divorced female, began treatment because of a fear of being alone. She had recently left her husband of many years and was considerably frightened about living by herself. A fundamental dynamic issue, conflict about dependency, was usually played out in her attachments to powerful, ungiving men. She characteristically idealized these individuals, but subsequently fled relationships when she felt herself becoming too dependent. During treatment, this pattern was recapitulated with the therapist. When he directed their combined attention to this development Ms. K. responded by becoming increasingly irresponsible with her monthly payments, an obvious acting out of her feelings. Though the therapist indicated that her mounting bill jeopardized their continued work, Ms. K. still could not control her finances, and treatment was ultimately terminated.
>
> Several months later Ms. K. settled her bill and asked to resume psychotherapy. The clinician agreed, but informed her that an important condition would be prompt payment of his fee. He also decided to positively reinforce her responsible behavior related to their financial interacton. He actively acknowledged timely payment of the bill, pointing out how it reflected her increased responsibility and autonomy, as well as a strengthened therapeutic alliance. Wishing to reinforce her more mature, independent functioning, he used specific comments and facial expressions to convey a definite sense of approval for her changed behavior whenever it was warranted. This facilitated the eventual examination of the conflict concerning her dependent yearnings. Ms. K. subsequently reported that she had engineered the earlier termination because of growing fear of the power she believed the therapist wielded over her. As treatment progressed, she developed an increasingly positive self-image, reflected in her considerably enhanced self-sufficiency.

Another application of learning theory to the limit setting process is negative reinforcement. A common example concerns seclusion of patients on an inpatient unit. As discussed in Chapter 4, the intervention carries a communication that an individual will be released from confinement only when he is able to demonstrate better control over his impulses. Combined with positive reinforcement, this intervention can help promote adaptive behaviors in patients. Negative reinforcement was also used during Ms. K.'s treatment, particularly when she threatened suicide as a seeming test of her doctor's resolve to support her independence. His initial response to her disturbing statements—increasing her medications and proposing extra therapy sessions—was followed by an escalation in her self-destructive behavior. As a result, he altered his therapeutic stance. He acknowledged how painful her feelings must be and informed her that she would have to admit herself to a hospital if she felt unable to control her impulses. He added that he would not meet with her while she was hospitalized, but would resume treatment upon her discharge. Following the imposition of these limits, her suicidal preoccupations abated. The therapist's attentive, but unflappable, attitude negatively reinforced Ms. K.'s self-destructive threats and ultimately allowed her to develop a more adaptive attitude toward her troubled emotions.

Learning via modeling frequently occurs when patients exceed established limits. Challenges to therapeutic authority often force clinicians to experience the same issues and conflicts that plague the patient. A common example concerns the individual's ability to act out in ways that make his caretakers experience the dysphoric affects he fears will overwhelm him. Individuals with borderline personality are particularly adept at provoking this response, often causing clinicians to feel an intense rage that mirrors the patient's internal make-up. Once this interaction is underway, the patient wittingly and unwittingly observes and evaluates how the therapist conducts himself. If he manages the particular issue via adequate limit setting, neither too overwhelming nor too austere to affect the patient's behavior, he provides an effective model for positive identification. In this manner, the patient learns more adaptive alternatives for expressing and controlling emotions. This occurred in Ms. K.'s treatment when the therapist provided a healthy model for dealing with regressive behavior by insisting on hospitalization should she be unable to control her impulses. Rather than becoming angry and disorganized, the therapist demonstrated that her behavior could be dealt with in a reasoned fashion different from her threatened method of conflict resolution. Modeling helped her appreciate that she, too, had the capacity to exercise more control over herself.

A common clinical situation that highlights the behavioral perspective of limit setting concerns treatment of a prototypically difficult patient, the disorganized individual. Disorganization occurs when organic or functional illness causes impaired cognition, judgment, and impulse control. Because the patient's ability to understand, remember, and, consequently, adhere to limits is greatly compromised, verbal negotiations are generally less successful than a learning approach. This is illustrated by the following vignette.

> Miss W., a middle-aged secretary, began treatment because of a long-standing depression. A bipolar disorder eventually emerged, marked by periods of paranoia and severe disorganization. During one such episode, the patient's usual regression in psychotherapy was aggravated by an increasing uncooperativeness with the entire treatment process. She became delinquent with her bill, appeared late for many sessions, failed to obtain necessary blood testing, and rapidly drifted into a deepening depression. Fearful of Miss W.'s self-destructive potential, her therapist was reluctant to terminate treatment. However, confrontation, clarification, and interpretation about the self-destructive behavior had no positive effect on her actions. He felt powerless and somewhat disorganized in his attempts to treat his contentious patient.
>
> Recognizing the ineffectiveness of discussing Miss W.'s decline, the clinician instituted a more behavioral approach to the limit setting. He informed the patient that he would not meet with her unless she paid for treatment at the start of each session. Surprisingly, she willingly complied with the requirement, as well as with several other conditions concerning her pharmacotherapy. The therapist praised her progress, which Miss W. obviously appreciated; however, she continued to distance herself via accusatory as well as self-denigrating comments. At one point she referred to her doctor's encouragement as "empty flattery" because "you just want my money." His incorrect response was to explore the statement in light of her long-standing pattern of unfulfilling relationships with men. Within a week, the patient's considerable disorganization recurred. Many of the previous

antitherapeutic behaviors reappeared, most likely in response to heightened transference feelings. The regression peaked when Miss W. called her therapist late one evening to announce that she could not keep the next day's appointment because of lack of funds. The clinician replied that unless she could pay him the following week he would have to permanently schedule another patient for their usual treatment hour. Though obviously furious, Miss. W. acknowledged that she understood her doctor's "conditions" and indicated she would see him in a week. The patient was organized and appropriate at the next meeting—she even paid in advance for the coming month's therapy. She continued to progress; however, it took several months before she could reflect back on the period and understand the unconscious issues, particularly her dependent yearnings, that contributed to her decline.

Miss W.'s case illustrates the importance of behavioral interventions in the limit setting process, particularly when a patient's maladaptive behaviors persist despite reasoned discussion. The individual's particular pathology, which may be an acute illness or a chronically ingrained characterologic issue, affects his cognitive processes in a way that prevents rational negotiation with the therapist. The presence of scattered or concretized thinking may seriously interfere with the patient's ability to understand abstract verbal interventions. Behavioral techniques must then become the mainstay of limit setting, until the patient is better able to discuss conflictual issues. In Miss W.'s case, several months passed before this evolution occurred; in fact, she regressed clinically because of her therapist's premature attempt to effect the shift.

CONCLUSION

Limit setting is most effective when the balance between its constituent theoretical components, the psychodynamic and the behavioral perspectives, is tailored to the patient's particular needs. By promoting self/non-self differentiation, therapeutic boundaries provide individuals with a clearer sense of their own identity, which becomes the fabric for healthier object relationships. This maturation process is achieved via intrapsychic change and conditioned learning.

By addressing deficits in ego functioning, limit setting helps overcome obstacles to adaptive functioning that derive from devel-

opmental difficulties. The psychodynamic mechanisms involved
pertain to the way the patient experiences affect, his difficulty expressing his drives, and the symptomatic and behavioral consequences of intrapsychic conflict. Therapeutic boundaries are also an
active demonstration by the clinician that there are alternatives to
the behaviors fostered by ineffectual parental models. By imposing
consistent, carefully conceived limits, which are neither excessive
nor negligent as to nurturing and control, he presents himself as a
more constant and caring individual than earlier authority figures in
the patient's life. This helps the patient give up his previous maladaptive behaviors and progressively adopt healthier patterns to guide
his interpersonal relationships.

REFERENCES

Berkowitz D: Vulnerability of the grandiose self and the psychotherapy of acting out. International Review of Psychoanalysis
4:13–21, 1977
Erickson E: The problem of ego identity. J Am Psychoanal Assoc
4:56–121, 1956
Frank J: Persuasion and Healing: A Comparative Study of Psychotherapy. Baltimore, Johns Hopkins University Press, 1961
Frosch J: Psychoanalytic considerations of the psychotic character. J
Am Psychoanal Assn 18:24–50, 1970
Goldberg R, Mann L, Wise T, et al: Parental qualities as perceived
by borderline personality disorders. The Hillside Journal of Clin-
ical Psychiatry 7(2):134–140, 1985
Hartmann H: Comments on the psychoanalytic theory of the ego,
in Essays on Ego Psychology. New York, International Universi-
ties Press, 1950, pp 113–141
Hartmann H: Notes on the superego. Psychoanal Study Child
16:42–81, 1962
Hartmann H, Kris B, Lowenstein R: Comments on the formation
of psychic structure. Psychoanal Study Child 2:11–18, 1946
Kernberg O: Borderline personality organization. J Am Psychoanal
Assoc 15:641–685, 1967
Kernberg O: A psychoanalytic classification of character pathology.

J Am Psychoanal Assoc 18:800–822, 1970
Kohut H: The Analysis of Self. New York, International Universities Press, 1971
Kohut H: Thoughts on narcissism and narcissistic rage. Psychoanal Study Child 27:360–401, 1972
Mahler M: A study of the separation–individuation process. Psychoanal Study Child 26:403–424, 1971
Mahler M, Pine F, Bergman A: The Psychological Birth of the Human Infant: Symbiosis and Individuation (Part II). New York, Basic Books, 1975
Skinner B: Science and Human Behavior. New York, MacMillan, 1953
Strayhorn J: Foundations of Clinical Psychiatry. Chicago, Year Book Medical Publishers, 1982

Chapter 3

Limit Setting
and the Transference
Relationship

*T*HE INTERACTION between patient and doctor is perceived
by many as a straightforward, if not mechanistic, occurrence. A
symptomatic individual presents himself for diagnosis and treatment with the expectation that he will either be made well or receive
significant relief. When his symptoms are most acute, and he is least
able to care for himself, the patient anticipates considerable support
from the physician, who for his part expects the individual's cooper-
ation and active participation in the therapeutic regimen. Most
individuals, physicians included, conceptualize the practice of medi-
cine in these terms—as a profession concerned with the rational
solution of problems. Obviously, considerable empathy and concern are involved in this process, since the particular problems under
consideration affect the physical and mental health of human
beings. However, treating illness is generally considered a cause-
and-effect intellectual exercise (as suggested by the biomedical
model) of determining etiology and prescribing the indicated therapeutic regimen. This is a parochial notion; considerably more tran-
spires when doctor and patient interact, though even a rudimentary

33

appreciation of this clinical phenomenology did not exist until the early 1900s.

Studies on Hysteria (Breuer and Freud 1893) was a germinal volume in the evolution of psychoanalysis, stimulating intense interest in such concepts as unconscious determinism and infantile sexuality. Probably its most significant contribution, however, concerned the recognition of powerful transference and countertransference reactions that characterize the doctor–patient relationship. The case of Anna O. was most notable in this regard. After being cured of her diverse psychosomatic symptoms, the patient developed a pseudocyesis and accused her physician, Josef Breuer, of siring the unborn child. His shock, fear, and outrage caused him to flee this unexplained situation. Freud, on the other hand, studied and deciphered the nature of Frau O.'s attachment to his colleague. The recent death of her father prompted the patient to compensate for that loss via a fantasied libidinal attachment to Dr. Breuer, an older man whose attentive efforts were reminiscent of prior parental concern. Moreover, biographical data suggest that Breuer's unconscious response to Anna O.'s incestuous feelings was heightened by his own oedipal wishes (Jones 1963). Though the intense feelings between Dr. Breuer and his patient were extreme examples of transference and countertransference phenomena, they reflect the ubiquitous nature of such distortions in the doctor–patient relationship—particularly during the course of a psychotherapy. Transference and countertransference feelings are often responsible for inappropriate interactions that may jeopardize the working alliance and significantly compromise the welfare of each member of the therapeutic relationship.

A century of study has yielded a comprehensive, sophisticated appreciation of the positive and negative aspects of the transference and countertransference. The powerful impact those emotions have on the psychotherapeutic work requires the clinician to work effectively with those feelings if treatment is to be successful. Helping the patient gain an interpersonal and experiential perspective on all transference distortions requires confrontation, clarification, and interpretation in insight-oriented work, and more concrete reality testing in supportive, anxiety-suppressive therapy. However, these interventions are not always successful in diffusing or therapeutically channeling the intense, irrational, sometimes dangerous emotions that make up the transference relationship. The effectiveness of all technical maneuvers depends on the ability of patient and physician to work collaboratively, an endeavor based on mutual trust. If the requisite motivation and commitment are lacking in either individual, the psychotherapy suffers. One consequence is escalating acting out by patients, whose maladaptive behaviors can affect the treatment process in the same fashion that Anna O.'s reactions to Dr. Breuer undermined their work. At such times, standard therapeutic maneuvers are usually ineffective. Continued acting out, and subsequent countertransference responses characterized by feelings of anxiety, helplessness, and rage, make active limit setting a necessity at this stage of a psychotherapy.

The basic philosophy of limit setting, as outlined in Chapter 1, is to contain and counteract maladaptive behaviors that so interfere with psychotherapy as to threaten its viability or the safety of the patient and/or therapist. This requires the clinician to first identify such behaviors to the patient and then delineate the limits to which therapy can withstand those actions. The final step is to clearly specify the consequences that will ensue should the patient ignore the explicitly detailed limits, consequences that include alteration of the treatment setting (for example, from outpatient to inpatient status), a change in therapists, or even termination of treatment. This chapter focuses on the relationship between transference distortions and the setting of limits, as well as countertransference reactions that may interfere with that process. However, transference and countertransference do not exist in a vacuum. Along with the working alliance and the phenomenon of acting out, they constitute the fundamental aspects of psychotherapy. Their interplay determines why, when, and how specific treatment interventions are made, because a change in any one of these entities—the prevailing transference and countertransference, the patient's acting out behaviors, and the status of the working alliance—affects and is subsequently affected by each of the other factors. As a consequence, setting limits on transference distortions that threaten the treatment can occur only by constantly monitoring the interaction of these four aspects of the psychotherapy. After the following definitions of each of the four components, three case histories are presented that illustrate the process of setting limits on transference distortions.

The Working Alliance

The working, or therapeutic, alliance is a particular type of object relationship existing between patient and therapist. Arising from the rational aspects of their interaction, it is the positive bond formed by the patient's conscious and unconscious desires to cooperate with the physician's conscious and unconscious efforts (Zetzel and Meissner 1973). It is basically a logical, nonneurotic communication between doctor and patient that serves as the analyzing and stabilizing factor for their other psychic interactions. As such, it is the essential prerequisite for the collaborative work of psychotherapy.

The working alliance requires specific contributions from each of its participants. The physician must present himself as a real person, inviting the patient's trust in his guidance, while simultaneously maintaining an objective, investigative posture. The patient must relate conscious and unconscious material in a relatively uncensored fashion, so as to progressively reveal his level of ego functioning and particular psychopathology. He must also exercise sufficient self-observation to appreciate and assess the psychologic conflicts and psychic defenses that manifest themselves in the clinical material, including his transference reactions. It is the latter characteristic that responds to the clinician's communicated dedication to the therapeutic task, with the result of achieving a working alliance. Essentially, the patient's "motivation to overcome his illness, his sense of helplessness, his conscious and rational willingness to cooperate, and his ability to follow instructions and insights" foster an identification with the therapist's attempts to uncover and understand the meaning and origin of emotional pain (Greenson 1967, p. 192).

Psychotherapy cannot occur in an environment lacking a viable working alliance. Not only is it an agreement between doctor and patient to work collaboratively, it is also an acknowledgment of their commitment to preserve the professional association even when it is threatened by events of the treatment. The working alliance helps to "resolve stresses, distortions and forces that would otherwise destroy it" (Meissner and Nicholi 1978, p. 359), such as extreme acting out behaviors. The greatest threat to a viable alliance usually comes from the patient who, lacking sufficient capacity for self-observation, may progressively transform the psychotherapy into an oppositional interaction. Increasingly active limit setting becomes necessary if the usual therapeutic maneuvers fail to abort such an impasse. The imposed therapeutic boundaries can take the form of directives concerning the process or content of the therapy. The former might involve a therapist's response to his patient's tardiness; the latter, direct challenges to extreme transference distortions.

Acting Out

Acting out is a process phenomenon that emanates from the interaction between patient and physician. In his early studies of psychoanalytic technique, Freud demonstrated that an individual's behavior within the treatment setting often expressed unstated emotions he harbored toward the therapist. He proposed that acting out one's feelings was ubiquitous and purposeful resistance to psychotherapy, antithetical to the *conversation* between patient and physician, which attempts to uncover underlying psychological issues. Moreover, Freud recognized that this powerful aspect of the psychotherapeutic process was a behavioral manifestation of some past event in an individual's life. His recognition of its compulsively repetitive quality suggested that such actions replay past occurrences in a disguised format. He postulated that this served the purpose of keeping those memories, and their associated affects, out of consciousness. In Freud's words, the patient represses by reproducing what he has forgotten "not as a memory but as an action; he *repeats* it, without, of course, knowing that he is repeating it." As an example, he describes how "the patient does not say that he remembers that he used to be defiant and critical towards his parents' authority; instead he behaves in that way to the doctor" (Freud 1914, p. 150).

Freud's initial perceptions about acting out have been progressively amended. This phenomenon is no longer considered to be exclusively confined to the treatment environment. Though the therapeutic relationship is the stimulus for these behaviors, patients frequently displace feelings for their physicians onto other people in their lives and act accordingly toward them. In addition, though the seemingly purposeful aspect of acting out suggests a component of rational control, it is now understood that the motivation for such behavior occurs outside the patient's consciousness. It is precisely for this reason that acting out poses a threat to the psychotherapeutic work. Merely understanding the origins of a patient's actions does not mean the clinician will be able to use that knowledge therapeutically, because individuals strenuously resist necessary insight via the very behaviors the clinician is attempting to contain. Vaillant (1977) underscores this point in his discussion of acting out as an immature ego mechanism frequently observed in patients undergoing psychotherapy. In order to relieve tension caused by postponement of instinctual expression, to avoid becoming consciously aware of the accompanying affect, patients directly express unconscious impulses via destructive behaviors such as self-inflicted injuries, impulsive acts, or alcohol and substance abuse. These actions often resist the standard therapeutic maneuvers, and consequently, limit setting becomes a necessary adjunctive intervention.

Transference

The transference is a distinctive type of object relationship, one determined by an individual's cathexes to important people in his past. It promotes unrealistic, sometimes irrational perceptions within the therapeutic environment, causing the patient to fight old ghosts perceived in the persona of the therapist. Greenson (1967) summarizes this clinical phenomenon as follows:

> Transference is the experiencing of feelings, drives, attitudes, fantasies, and defenses toward a person in the present which do not befit that person but are a repetition of reactions originating in regard to significant persons of early childhood, unconsciously displaced onto figures in the present. (p. 155)

Transference has a twofold role in the psychotherapeutic process. First, it is a window into the past and thus the unconscious. By studying recurrent interactions between the patient and himself, the therapist progressively learns of experiences that produced the former's emotional distress. He comes to understand the patient's unacknowledged emotions, his difficulty dealing with them over the years, and the symptomatic and behavioral compromises made to offset those painful feelings. In this regard, the transference is the foundation of both supportive and insight-oriented psychotherapy. The structure and reassurance provided by the former is greatly facilitated by the therapist's comprehensive understanding of the various identifications that positively and negatively influence his patient. As for anxiety-provoking psychodynamic psychotherapy, the transference is the clinician's Rosetta stone for deciphering unconscious material. He uses this key to help the patient acknowledge, bear, and put into perspective those painful affects that adversely affect his functioning and thus his happiness (Semrad 1969). Although the therapeutic significance of the transference became apparent when psychoanalysis was first being studied and elaborated as a treatment modality (Freud evolved his thesis concerning the transference neurosis in his classic case studies [1893, 1905, 1918], developed it in his early papers on technique [1914, 1915], and refined it in later works [1937]), utilization of the transference is not confined to traditional psychoanalytic work. It is the cornerstone of long-term, insight-oriented psychotherapy, as well as the technique advocated by contemporary brief psychotherapists (Sifneos 1972; Malan 1976; Davanloo 1980).

In contrast to its facilitating role, transference is also a powerful resistance. By causing an individual to react to the therapist as if he were someone other than the treating physician, transference may so compromise the patient's observing ego that he loses the ability to effectively reality test many of his perceptions. This can negate the therapist's positive influence in supportive work, and prevent attainment of meaningful insight in the case of psychodynamic psychotherapy. Unresolved transference may even bring treatment to a permanent halt by causing the patient to flee an intensely uncomfortable therapeutic environment characterized by extremely inappropriate affects that span the spectrum from murderous rage to limitless love to infantile helplessness.

The transference can make for the best and the worst of times in psychiatric treatment. To paraphrase Greenson, it is an instrument of irreplaceable value, as well as the source of greatest danger. Maximizing its facilitating role while simultaneously containing its antitherapeutic impact is one of the physician's most exacting tasks. Though never wholly accountable for the success of a psychotherapy, it is his clear responsibility to recognize the need for limit setting when his usual interventions are ineffective in resolving those transference distortions that threaten treatment. At these times, he must reemphasize to the patient a fundamental tenet of treatment: All transference feelings are appropriate for discussion, but their expression in ways that endanger the psychotherapeutic process must cease if treatment is to continue.

Countertransference

Though generally understood as those unconscious attitudes of the therapist that interfere with treatment, countertransference actually has several defined meanings (Little 1951). Reich's (1951) understanding of this clinical phenomenon is both comprehensive and clinically directed. In her words,

> Countertransference thus comprises the effects of the analyst's own unconscious needs and conflicts on his understanding or technique. In such cases the patient represents for the analyst an object of the past on to whom past feelings and wishes are projected, just as it happens in the patient's transference situation with the analyst. The provoking factor for such an occurrence may be something in the patient's personality or material or something in the analytic situation as such. (p. 26)

Implied in this definition are the concepts of "acute" and "chronic" forms of countertransference, which Reich likens respectively to "incidental hysterical symptoms in contrast to permanent character disorders" (p. 28). With the former, a particular issue arising in treatment may suddenly trigger unconscious forces within the therapist that cloud clinical neutrality. This often derives from identification with the patient, possibly stemming from a shared life experience. A chronically ingrained countertransference can derive from the therapist's inappropriate response to a patient who reminds him of a significant person from his own past, or from the therapeutic situation itself, which may adversely affect the clinician because of some unresolved character pathology. An example of the latter situation involves "unconscious aggression [which] may cause the analyst to be over-conciliatory, hesitant and unable to be firm when necessary" (Reich 1951, p. 27). Greenson (1967) discusses how these situations can produce insidious, persistent antitherapeutic results because of the therapist's constant misreading of clinical material.

Negative countertransference is acted out because of the physician's need to maintain *his* emotional equilibrium. As a result, he may (consciously or unconsciously) communicate a desire to avoid certain issues in treatment. The patient can act out, in turn, by (consciously or unconsciously) shutting off important clinical material in response to his therapist's unstated request. Therapy thus becomes self-contradictory, as the patient becomes the clinician's caretaker. More severe instances of negative countertransference can endanger patients; for example, inattention to stated self-destructive urges might cause a seriously depressed individual to flee therapy, in the extreme case by suicide. Negative countertransference not only precipitates clinical regression in this fashion, it also accelerates decline by compromising the therapist's ability to effectively set limits. Unable to appreciate his own contribution to a therapeutic impasse, the clinician may become increasingly frustrated with the patient's presumed resistance. Persistent overt and covert demands for clinical improvement simply aggravate the patient's regression, which then heightens the therapist's resentment. Effective limit setting is not possible in such an environment.

That the description of countertransference conjures up thoughts of the transference is not surprising; the two phenomena are intricately intertwined. And, like the facilitating role of the transference, the countertransference also has its positive side. The very process of absorbing the clinical material requires the therapist to infuse his own unconscious into the treatment situation. Freud discussed this when advocating listening to the patient with free-floating, as well as studied, attention. The therapeutic screen is not just a neutral target for the patient's projected unconscious. Though the stepwise understanding of his fears, wishes, and needs demands objectivity and studied judgment on the part of the therapist, it also requires an interaction between the two participants on an unstructured, unconscious level. The therapist's countertransference can foster the so-called "good therapeutic match" if his unconscious issues complement those of the patient. For example, a clinician with well-sublimated aggressive urges is better equipped to avoid an individual's attempts to engage him in distracting, ennervating struggles. This allows the two of them to more stringently adhere to the therapeutic task of focusing on the psychic origins of the patient's competitiveness, in order to work through the associated feelings.

Countertransference can be used in a more active manner to facilitate treatment. Just as psychotherapy helps a patient retrieve repressed material by bringing it to preconscious and conscious levels of awareness, it can have a similar effect on the therapist's psyche. His gradual comprehension of countertransference feelings provides him with material that can be judiciously shared with the patient. These so-called countertransference interpretations can benefit the therapy in several ways. First, the patient's tendency to idealize the therapist is limited; the physician becomes less of a distant, omniscient figure and more of a human being capable of emotional give and take. This enhances the patient's sense of independence and thereby facilitates the collaborative work of therapy. Second, the patient receives feedback concerning his impact on people. In this manner, the therapy provides knowledge about his intrapsychic functioning, as well as valuable information concerning his interpersonal relationships. Finally, by recognizing and sharing countertransference feelings with his patient, the therapist is less likely to act out those emotions in a counterproductive manner.

In sum, countertransference is an integral part of insight-oriented and supportive psychotherapy that can either benefit or harm the patient and/or therapist. This is underscored in Little's (1951) general description of the therapeutic interaction:

> Unconscious elements can be both normal and pathological, and not all repression is pathological any more than all conscious elements are "normal." The whole patient–analyst relationship includes both "normal" and pathological, conscious and unconscious, transference and counter-transference, in varying proportions; it will always include something which is specific to both the individual patient and the individual analyst. (p. 33)

Case Examples

The continuous interaction of these fundamental aspects of psychotherapy—the working alliance, acting out behaviors, transference, and countertransference—defines the focus, rhythm, and progress of treatment. Their interplay determines whether therapy is primarily work oriented or is a regressive, nonproductive endeavor. The standard therapeutic maneuvers are usually sufficient to negotiate this interaction; however, active limit setting becomes necessary when an individual's level of resistance far exceeds his motivation for improvement. In this circumstance, the clinician attempts to productively refocus the collaborative work of psychotherapy by imposing therapeutic boundaries and delineating the consequences for ignoring those guidelines. The goal is to minimize maladaptive acting out behaviors in order to facilitate verbal expression and the working through of underlying affects within the safety of the treatment setting.

The following case histories illustrate the adverse impact of extreme transference distortions, indicating how they affect the other parameters of treatment in ways which threaten the psychotherapy. Case One details the consequences when a patient splits off negative transference feelings from the treatment and indiscriminately acts them out with various people in his life. Case Two illustrates excessive dependency in the transference relationship and the emergence of excessive anger when that dependency is not satisfied. Case Three demonstrates the need for limit setting with an overly positive transference, in this instance one that is highly erotized. Though the clinical material has been divided according to a predominant type of transference reaction, it should be emphasized that most clinical situations are not that clear-cut. The transference is frequently disguised and consequently deceptive, such as when a large component of hostility underlies extreme dependency or suspiciousness.

Case One

Michael, a 19-year-old office worker, began treatment because of anxiety and excessive fatigue. His symptoms interfered with work and his social relationships, and he was beginning to fear that they would progress to the point where "I won't be able to go out at all." He dated the onset of symptoms to the end of a relationship with a co-worker, a woman who welcomed his friendship but not his sexual advances. As this was his first attempt at a sexual relationship, her rejection was a considerable narcissistic affront to Michael. Although a handsome young man, he became preoccupied with doubts about his attractiveness to women, and despite the fact that he had never experienced homosexual feelings he began to wonder if he was " a latent fag." These ruminations were accompanied by generalized anxiety, as well as specific fears that relatives and friends would ridicule him for failing to win "a serious girlfriend." His daily functioning declined, prompting several warnings from his employer and causing him to progressively withdraw from the world. Spending increasing amounts of time in his room, he began to think he was "going crazy" when he twice heard a man's voice call him "a total loser." At that point he sought psychiatric treatment.

Following a series of diagnostic interviews, and a complete neurologic work-up, Michael was diagnosed as suffering from an adjustment disorder with anxiety and depressive symptoms. He was noted to have passive–dependent personality traits; however, the presence of more serious character pathology, specifically, a borderline personality disorder, was considered. Recommended treatment included twice-weekly individual psychotherapy, primarily supportive in nature, and low-dose neuroleptic medication. He responded well to this regimen; he formed a strong, positive attachment to his therapist, Dr. C., and realized considerable and rapid symptomatic relief. Dysthymia became the primary working diagnosis when Michael became more depressed as his anxiety remitted. At that point, therapy was directed toward the uncovering of psychodynamic and psychogenetic material and focused less on recent events. The patient made this transition with seeming ease and readily revealed pertinent anamnestic data.

The youngest of two brothers, Michael had grown up in a tumultuous household. His alcoholic father was legally prevented from residing with his family when the patient was 11, due to repeated physical assaults on his wife and children. Michael's mother subsequently obtained a divorce and moved the family to another city, a difficult transition for the patient. Uprooted from a school he enjoyed, and removed from a peer group that respected him as a leader, Michael felt alienated and lonely in his new environment. He resented the separation from his extended family and felt even more neglected when his mother began full-time work for the first time. This feeling was heightened when she remarried shortly after the patient's 13th birthday. Although his stepfather was a caring man, affording Michael the same attention and concern he directed toward his own sons, the patient felt uneasy at home. He disliked both of his older stepbrothers, because "they made fun of me and sometimes beat me up." He also bristled at his stepfather's strictness, constantly afraid that his discipline would progress to the abuse he had received from his biologic father. Michael's new life situation left him feeling lonely, resentful, and anxious; however, he never shared these emotions, fearing persecution or retaliation if he voiced his discontents. He secretly planned to leave home and make his own happiness as soon as he was self-sufficient. He felt he was progressing toward that goal when he developed his presenting symptoms.

While relating his history, Michael showed steady clinical improvement. Specific themes were identified by Dr. C., and the patient demonstrated an ability to work through feelings associated with numerous episodes that highlighted those issues. For example, his life was rife with repeated rejections and losses, most recently the one involving his co-worker. In the course of several therapy sessions he effectively grieved her, progressing through identifiable affective stages that culminated in considerable resolution of his many feelings. Michael investigated other past and present relationships that had caused him distress, attaining an appropriate emotional perspective on most of them. His psychotherapy progressed well, except for a particular dimension of the treatment that was disturbing to Dr. C.: The patient essentially ignored the transference relationship. He minimized or denied obvious parallels between his feelings toward people in his past or current life and those for Dr. C. The very few times he addressed the transference it was to praise his doctor for "helping me get back on track." Though pleased with Michael's clinical progress, Dr. C. was distressed by the absence of any negative transference. His concern was heightened when it became necessary to terminate therapy prematurely due to an unanticipated move. Michael's psychodynamics rendered him particularly vulnerable to the unexpected loss of his physician, yet he acted calmly to the announced termination. He repeatedly denied negative feelings about the event, spent the concluding meetings voicing appreciation for his doctor's help, and expressed confidence about the future. Though Michael remained clinically stable throughout this period, Dr. C. felt that his psychotherapy was incomplete despite their five months of work together. Consequently, he suggested that Michael continue in treatment, which the patient agreed to, and transfer to another doctor was arranged.

Michael began regressing shortly after the transition to his new therapist, Dr. R. His job performance began to decline, prompting criticism from his supervisor. Michael spent several therapy sessions complaining about his superior's unreasonableness, arbitrariness, and stupidity, as tension between the two of them developed into increasingly bitter arguments. His discontent soon appeared at home. Resentment of his stepfather's rigidity caused Michael, for the first time, to openly complain about certain family decisions. His stepfather responded by asserting even greater control, which further provoked the patient. Michael also attempted to initiate a relationship with an obviously unavailable woman and was furious when his advances were rebuked. As he related each setback to his new therapist, Michael expressed increasing doubts about the utility of treatment.

Dr. R. interpreted his patient's decline as a manifestation of unstated anger toward both of his therapists. He felt that Michael was furious at Dr. C. for leaving and that his regression was the expression of that anger, a demonstration that little had been accomplished during their work together. Moreover, Michael's behavior was also an angry demand that his new therapist do something to halt the decline. Dr. R. suggested that Michael's inability or unwillingness to openly acknowledge and discuss the hostility he felt toward his therapists caused him to displace those feelings onto people in his life, which was reflected in his self-defeating behavior. Dr. R. emphasized that his office was the appropriate arena for discussing, understanding, and thereby controlling Michael's current feelings. He suggested that they begin by exploring his reaction to Dr. C.'s departure; if he could work through the feelings precipitated by that loss, those emotions would no longer interfere with his daily functioning. While politely rejecting this hypothesis, Michael could hardly disguise his obvious anger and contempt for Dr. R. He reported, "You can only be guessing how I feel towards people because you really don't understand me well enough yet." Not only did his regression continue, his anger became increasingly dangerous. Fearing that he would "explode" following an incident with his stepfather, Michael slashed the family cat with a penknife after the animal had scratched him. During the next two days, he was preoccupied with ruminations about stabbing his stepfather, feelings he reported to Dr. R. during their next meeting. At the same time he announced that he would soon be discontinuing treatment because "it hasn't really helped me at all."

The usual therapeutic maneuvers were clearly ineffective in dealing with Michael 's anger, which had escalated to potentially lethal proportions. His overdetermined reaction to the loss of Dr. C., matched by an equally overdetermined effort to deny his rage and sense of abandonment, caused him to act out his aggression in an almost indiscriminate manner. The therapeutic impasse, aggravated by a growing potential for violence, necessitated the rapid implementation of therapeutic boundaries. Dr. R. envisioned two specific goals of limit setting. First, the treatment environment had to be made safe enough for the patient to feel secure in verbalizing emotions, particularly his aggressive feelings. Next, opportunities for acting out transference feelings outside the therapeutic setting had to be severely restricted, in order to protect Michael and the people in his life from his maladaptive behaviors. With these goals in mind, Dr. R. instituted the following limit setting interventions.

First, Michael was hospitalized. He accepted this action only after being threatened with involuntary commitment, despite his recognition that interaction with the people in his daily environment caused a dysphoric turmoil that made him uncomfortable and dangerous. His resistance to hospitalization rapidly subsided as he felt increasingly secure in the structured routine, and he responded to a short course of tranquillizing medications. Considerably calmer, he began "feeling like my old self" and was no longer worried about his emotions "getting out of control."

Next, in an effort to diminish the destructive feuding at home, a series of twice-weekly family meetings commenced. These included all members of the household and were initially structured as problem-solving exercises focused on conflict resolution. Specific behavioral regimens were then formulated to implement at the outset of any family argument. Though these strategies proved useful while Michael was hospitalized, their utility after discharge remained uncertain. Consequently, the family meetings also explored possible alternative living arrangements as a means of avoiding the tensions at home.

Third, the turmoil at Michael's job had to subside. Dr. R. indicated that the patient could exercise several options regarding his employment, which included making peace with his supervisor, requesting a proposed transfer within the office, or simply leaving the job. Though the decision was left entirely up to the patient, Dr. R. did reserve the right to contact Michael's employer after discharge in order to monitor his work situation. This was acceptable to the patient, who had actually requested such contact when he was initially hospitalized.

The final limit concerned solely the psychotherapeutic work. Detailing his thoughts about Michael's decompensation, Dr. R. offered the opinion that the patient felt considerable hostility toward his first therapist because of his unplanned departure. Michael characteristically inhibited that anger because of feared retaliation, an interpersonal style that mirrored his relationship with his biologic father. Dr. R. explained that Michael's efforts to protect both therapists from his fury reflected this central, and exceedingly detrimental, psychodynamic issue. He again described how the patient had so neutralized his anger within the therapeutic setting that it overflowed into the relationships of his daily life, resulting in the many skirmishes at home and in the workplace. Consequently, while Michael was hospitalized the primary focus of their psychotherapeutic work would be an exploration of Michael's feelings toward his first therapist. Dr. R. made it clear that he would continually guide treatment toward that end. Reminding the patient that he had already demonstrated his capacity to effectively grieve for the female co-worker who rejected him, Dr. R. expressed his belief that Michael could achieve a similarly positive resolution to his association with Dr. C. Dr. R. stressed that this was the only way for the patient to learn how to express anger in a constructive fashion without becoming uncontrollably angry or fearful of provoking one's sadistic retaliation. He emphasized that he would begin every therapy hour by asking the patient to discuss Dr. C. and would interrupt whenever Michael wandered from that topic. Dr. R. felt that such an approach would mobilize the patient's anger toward both of his therapists.

Following the imposition of therapeutic boundaries, which combined behavioral principles with psychodynamically oriented psychotherapy, the patient began to improve dramatically. The external limits evolved into his growing sense of internal control; he recognized that concerns about the effects of his anger were more fantasy than fact and consequently began addressing the negative transference. He ventilated criticism, disappointment, and sadness for Dr. C., while retaining positive feelings for him. During two subsequent years of treatment, a similar process occurred with Dr. R. The patient's ability to openly discuss distressing transference feelings, instead of acting them out with the various individuals who populated his daily life, made for a happier, more productive existence. Michael eventually reached a relative peace with his stepfather and functioned more independently within the family, even if that meant disagreement between the two of them. His job performance improved, earning him two impressive promotions, and he soon became engaged. By preventing the patient from splitting off the negative transference from the therapeutic environment, limit setting had effectively controlled Michael's self-defeating behavior of indiscriminate expression of emotions. This preserved the psychotherapy and ultimately enabled him to make significant gains in his life.

Case Two

Lynne K., a 23-year-old secretary, was brought to the emergency room in the throes of a severe anxiety attack. She had been awakened in the middle of the night by "a terrible pounding in my chest," and was convinced she was "dying from a heart attack." Her frightened screams prompted neighbors to call the police, who took her to the hospital. Although examination confirmed her good physical health, reassurance failed to alleviate Miss K.'s terror. She ultimately required sedation and spent the remainder of the night asleep on a stretcher. She awoke feeling calm and composed and dismissed suggestions that her symptoms had been emotionally based. However, after identical episodes during each of the following three nights she consented to a psychiatric consultation.

Miss K. was evaluated by Dr. T. in the outpatient department a week after her first anxiety attack. She had been asymptomatic for several nights and, as a result, reported that she felt "the worst is over." She was indifferent and removed when asked about anxiety symptoms; she minimized the obvious terror and somatic distress she had experienced and became increasingly vague and guarded when pressed to discuss her attacks. She felt that "talking about it may bring them back." On the other hand, she was quite willing to relate her tragic life history, which was rife with trauma and despair.

When she was four, Lynne K.'s mother was discovered to have metastatic breast cancer. The diagnosis was made at the time she delivered her second child, Miss K.'s younger brother. Extensive and debilitating treatment failed to arrest her disease; she had a progressive downhill course over a three-and-a-half-year period and died on her daughter's eighth birthday. Lynne K. told the consulting psychiatrist she "couldn't imagine a worse way to start life . . . being a young girl and watching your mother die piece by piece." Her sorrows were multiple. Naturally there was the obvious fear and anguish from witnessing her mother in severe pain, wasting away, progressively losing control of her mental and physical functioning. Miss K. recalled "sitting with my mother all day long" during her final weeks, "even though she didn't know who I was." She also remembered being "neglected" by her father. She claimed to have understood his preoccupation with a dying spouse, as well as his responsibilities to his younger child, "who needed the attention more than I did." Nevertheless, she resented her father's distance. During the course of her mother's illness, Miss K. felt "there was no one there for me." The final cruelty in her young life occurred a year later when her father died suddenly of a heart attack just after her birthday. The patient and her brother were taken in by an elderly aunt and uncle who she regarded as "kind, concerned and loving." They provided material and emotional support and, according to Miss K., were largely responsible for her intellectual development and educational success. However, because of their age, and the fact that they never raised children of their own, she felt "they just didn't know enough to be adequate parents." In her opinion, the chronic unhappiness she experienced throughout her adolescence and early adult life was "inevitable because I was an orphan by age nine."

Despite these severe hardships, Miss K. had never previously experienced emotional symptoms that warranted psychiatric intervention. Consequently, she was perplexed by her anxiety attacks, particularly because she could not identify any precipitating stress. That, plus the absence of symptoms for three nights, suggested to her that the episodes were due to an undiagnosed physical ailment.

She was amused by the psychiatrist's suggestion that the stresses of her earlier life might be connected with her current attacks. She dismissed the hypothesis, implying that he was trying to cover up for the other physicians' inability to correctly diagnose her illness. She discarded as "coincidence" the fact that her attacks began the week of her birthday—an emotionally charged time of the year for her—and that she initially interpreted her palpitations as a fatal heart attack, the cause of her father's demise. After talking with the consultant for an hour, Miss K. requested "the name of a good internist, someone who could get to the bottom of this."

Miss K.'s attacks continued over the next year, during which time she invested considerable time, energy, and money with numerous physicians in an attempt to determine what she believed to be a physical etiology for her symptoms. A common pattern developed between the patient and her doctors. After a careful history and examination, each informed her that she was suffering from excessive anxiety. She rejected these pronouncements out of hand, badgered each clinician to perform some sophisticated diagnostic procedure, and was repeatedly angered when the tests proved normal. She then cajoled each doctor to prescribe various cardiac medications, usually beta-blockers, some of which provided short-term relief, but never lasting improvement. Eventually, she reluctantly followed the advice of these physicians and recontacted Dr. T. She expressed a desire "to further discuss the possible connection between my emotions and my attacks." After an extended evaluation he believed that Miss K.'s anxiety attacks represented a pathological grief reaction to the deaths of her parents. He also diagnosed a chronic dysthymia and felt that individual psychotherapy and a concurrent trial of an anxiolytic agent were indicated. Tricyclic antidepressant medication was considered as a therapeutic alternative.

While informing Miss K. of the treatment recommendations, Dr. T. also began to educate her as to the psychotherapeutic process. He particularly stressed the need to *talk* about distressing feelings, expressing concern about her proclivity toward action when stressed. He described their work as collaborative, discounted any claims to omnipotence, and promised no quick cures. The patient seemed receptive to his directives, save those concerning medications. She wanted no part of "pills that make me look and act like a zombie," and adamantly refused them. Dr. T. did not press the issue, but indicated that he would do so if he felt she required medications to maintain an acceptable level of functioning. Miss K. said she understood his thinking, and agreed to twice-weekly meetings.

The following morning, the patient called to confirm her appointment times. Dr. T. returned the call at the end of the work day, at which time Miss K. told him she had "worried all day that he wasn't going to call back." Dr. T. remarked that they could explore those concerns when they next met and reminded her of the designated time. Later that evening the patient again phoned, inquiring if Dr. T. had been annoyed by her earlier call. Instead of directly responding to the question he said they could discuss whatever was on her mind during her appointment the following day. He also reminded her that his patients could contact him after office hours only during an emergency. Sounding contrite, Miss K. ended the brief conversation.

Several hours later, Dr. T. was awakened by a call from a local emergency room physician. He was informed that his patient had just come to the hospital in a "state of total panic" pleading with the intern to "call my doctor right away because he knows all about my condition." Miss K.'s behavior represented a disturbingly clear statement of her excessive dependency, her wish to abdicate responsibility for her welfare to the therapist she hoped would magically cure her. Appreciating the malignant potential of this dependency, Dr. T. recognized the necessity of rapidly imposing therapeutic boundaries on his patient's behavior. Consequently, he advised the emergency room physician as to acute treatment of the patient's anxiety, but left the decision about disposition entirely up to the house officer. Dr. T. asked that Miss K. be reminded of her appointment the next day, adding that she should contact him to reschedule if she required admission to the hospital. He ended the conversation by stating that he would not treat Miss K. as an inpatient, but would gladly talk with the staff physician assigned her case. Dr. T. returned to sleep wondering if the psychotherapy with his new patient had ended before formally beginning.

The next morning Miss K. appeared for her appointment disheveled, distraught, and several minutes late. Her announced purpose for coming was to personally inform Dr. T. of his insensitivity and incompetence "as a psychiatrist and a human being." She was incredulous that he could have "acted so cold"; she felt "completely abandoned," particularly after he had "promised to help get rid of my anxiety." She ended her critical discourse by stating that his inaction the previous evening had not only proved he could "not be trusted," but also suggested to her that he "knew all along my problem was a physical one." When she was finished, Dr. T. said that he wanted to relate his understanding of her recent behavior, and asked if she was interested in hearing his thoughts. She did not respond to the question. He repeated it, adding that he would not be offended if she chose to leave, but as her appointment was not yet over he was willing to share his ideas about the previous evening. Her continued silence prompted Dr. T. to reiterate the alternatives —Miss K. could leave the office, they could sit in silence for the remaining few minutes, or he would relate his thinking about her behavior to date. Miss K. begrudgingly agreed to the latter course. Believing that this would be his only opportunity to convince his patient of the need for psychiatric treatment, Dr. T. was comforting and comprehensive in relating his understanding of her chronic emotional pain. His threefold approach entailed clarifying central psychodynamic issues, illustrating their operation in the transference relationship, and setting appropriate limits on behaviors that threatened the viability of treatment.

To begin with, Dr. T. underscored to Miss K. how exquisitely sensitive she was to rejection or perceived neglect. Excluding the first four years of her life, she had been severely deprived of parental attention. Her mother's illness caused a growing distance between her and her mother as well as between her and her father who was preoccupied with his own grief while struggling to care for two young children. With his death, the patient was suddenly and thoroughly denied the love and protection of her parents. By age nine she had suffered the extreme emotional pain of their abandonment and learned the harsh reality that life holds no guarantees. The impact on her subsequent development was considerable: It contributed to a lifelong characterologic trait of excessive dependency in her object relationships. Having been deprived the guidance and support of her parents while she was developing the skills and maturity of more autonomous functioning, she ferociously attempted to ensure that her dependency needs would always be fulfillled in all her interpersonal relationships. Obviously, this was a self-defeating style that consistently alienated the many people in her life to whom she had abdicated responsibility for her welfare. Many exploited Miss K.'s weakness, using her to satisfy their own need for power and control. All eventually tired of their role as protector; when they ended the association with the patient, it prompted her to immediately and frantically search for someone else who would make her feel safe and secure. When this behavior was no longer able to satisfy the intense feelings of fear and anger associated with each abandonent, she effected a compromise between her underlying affects and a defense against those emotions via her anxiety symptoms. Dr. T. told Miss K. that her attacks were an expression of her rage for having lost her parents as a young child and for being constantly frustrated in her efforts to secure a guaranteed substitute for the nurturing she never really had. Moreover, he suggested that she could never make up for their loss, that all her attempts to do so had driven people away and actually intensified her feelings of abandonment, and that her primary goal in therapy would be to grieve for her parents—a task she had never completed.

After detailing these unconscious motivations to his patient, Dr. T. emphasized that those same forces seemed to have already pervaded their relationship. He interpreted the unnecessary calls as unstated communications of her neediness, messages that put him on notice as to how much she required attention. He proposed that her latest anxiety attack was an expression of anger, specifically directed at him for admonishing her about the phone calls, as well as globally directed in payment for a life of real and perceived rejections. Most important, Dr. T. felt that the events of the previous 24 hours had clearly indicated that each of them had different goals for the psychotherapy: He wished to help her effectively grieve her parents, thereby freeing her from the self-destructive life-style of pathologic dependency; she wished to use their therapeutic relationship exclusively to satisfy her dependent wishes. Dr. T. suggested that if the latter alternative prevailed Miss K. would only succeed in engaging him as she had numerous other protectors. She would initially idealize him, perceiving him as the panacea for her lifelong distress, and then denigrate him after he caused her some disappointment or frustration. Ultimately, she would leave treatment feeling angry and cheated, again having learned little about the shared intimacy and interdependence characteristic of a mature relationship. Wishing to prevent this scenario, Dr. T. said that he would insist on certain rules concerning the psychotherapy if Miss K. chose to continue treatment. He then proceeded to detail the therapeutic boundaries.

To begin with, Dr. T. insisted on limited phone contact between the two of them, requesting that Miss K. not call in between appointments. He acknowledged the terror and foreboding she experienced with each attack, as well as the reassurance she might realize merely by talking with him. However, he felt such interaction would be generally detrimental to her welfare, since the long-term effect of enhancing her dependency would offset any short-term relief. In addition, he reported that excessive phone contact would be burdensome and would stir his own feelings of anger and resentment. Under those circumstances their therapeutic relationship would simply degenerate into a recapitulation of the pathologic object relationships that characterized her daily life. When asked what to do "in an emergency," Dr. T. replied that the events of the previous evening demonstrated to him that she could care for herself in that circumstance.

Next, the role of medications was discussed. Though he wanted to assess the effects of an anxiolytic agent, Dr. T. temporized for two reasons. First, given Miss K.'s adamant opposition to psychoactive drugs, he felt it would enhance the therapeutic alliance if she felt she retained control over that issue. Second, he wished to observe her response to psychotherapy. Consequently, he did not insist on medication, but indicated he would do so if her anxiety attacks increased in frequency and/or severity. Given her character pathology, he was privately concerned about her potential for abusing medications. However, he was prepared to offer a pill that might reduce Miss K.'s level of symptomatic distress, as well as serve as a transitional object to him; on balance, he judged that level of dependency preferable to the one she was currently attempting to effect.

Third, Dr. T. felt that a concrete description concerning his degree of availability was a crucial therapeutic boundary that needed to be established at this point in their relationship. He reiterated the proposed appointment times, described how he alternated weekend coverage with colleagues, and discussed his projected schedule for the next few months, including vacations and professional commitments that would interfere with their planned meetings. He indicated his policy of rescheduling such appointments whenever possible, as well as those that either one of them could not attend because of illness. Finally, he observed that Miss K. began every relationship with conscious and unconscious fears that her partner would depart unexpectedly, leaving her saddened, lonely, and defenseless. Therefore he felt it necessary to state that to his knowledge he was in good health and his physical condition should not have an adverse impact on his ability to work with her. Further, he informed her that he had no plans of relocating or moving to another city. Dr. T. concluded by saying that he had related to Miss K. all relevant information concerning his professional availability and that he anticipated no further questions concerning the subject. He specifically stated that phone calls like the ones she had made the previous evening were unacceptable to him.

Dr. T. was well aware that setting the above limits at this stage of treatment carried considerable risk. Miss K.'s predominant feelings toward him were negative, and the working alliance was at best tenuous. However, given her stated desire to terminate therapy because of his alleged insensitivity, he felt he had to proceed in this fashion. Before Dr. T. could help his patient reality test her transference distortions she had to stop acting out those feelings in ways that merely reenforced her maladaptive dependency. In an attempt to maximize his chance for success, Dr. T. prefaced the limit setting with clear clarifications and interpretations concerning his patient's feelings and behavior. Yet he was not greatly surprised when she reiterated her intention to discontinue treatment "because my problem is a physical one and you just don't understand that." He restated his belief that her anxiety attacks represented a physical response to unresolved emotions caused by losses she had experienced during her life and concluded the meeting by asking her to think about what they had discussed. He invited her to contact him if she changed her mind about therapy.

Several weeks later, Dr. T. was surprised by a phone call from Miss K. in which she announced her wish "to resume psychotherapy." She offered no reason for this decision, and was guarded and vague when pressed for one during their subsequent meeting. Eventually reporting she had "researched Dr. T.," she acknowledged being "extremely impressed by his professional credentials." She therefore concluded that he "was probably right about my attacks" and presented herself for "definitive treatment." When asked to explain that term she responded by saying she anticipated "a complete cure." At this point, Dr. T. repeated that he was willing to work with Miss K. toward that end, but felt it necessary to highlight what he interpreted as a pathologically motivated aspect of her decision to recontact him. He pointed out how her "research" had fostered an idealized image of him, resulting in unfounded expectations such as "a complete cure." He indicated that this was a repetition of her old pattern; she was disguising her overwhelming dependency, her wish to be cared for and protected, with a rationalization about his presumed expertise. Consequently, whereas he wholeheartedly believed that she required psychiatric treatment, he wanted to state specifically that the success of their future work depended much more on collaborative effort than on his clinical abilities and experience. He could not guarantee the results of psychotherapy, and, of course, if she resumed treatment he would insist on the therapeutic boundaries he had previously detailed.

Though visibly annoyed over what she referred to as Dr. T.'s habit of "seeing dependency in everything I do," Miss K. agreed to treatment. Why she ultimately made that commitment was never clear to her physician. Since the psychotherapy proceeded with much less difficulty than expected, however, he was willing to live with that uncertainty. Although the early weeks were characterized by considerable testing of therapeutic boundaries, Miss K.'s acting out progressively diminished. After a tentative beginning, she became absorbed in grieving her parents; symptomatic improvement paralleled this course, and she was essentially free of anxiety attacks approximately six months into the treatment. She regressed periodically, lapsing into relative degrees of helplessness and dependency when stressed by events in her life. At those times, she frequently infused her fear and disappointment into the transference, but was generally able to work through those feelings. Her most significant regressions occurred when she was actually deprived of Dr. T., particularly during his vacations. However, she effectively dealt with these episodes via grief work focused on feelings of loss caused by his absences. In addition, these periods produced her first insights into the hostile component of her acting out behaviors.

Attention to this crucial aspect of her psychodynamics eventually permitted a healthy termination of treatment. Miss K.'s association with Dr. T. was the first important relationship in her life that ended without her feeling depleted, helpless, and despairing of the future. Though she felt deprived of a caring friend, she clearly recognized her ability to function effectively without requiring his support. This realization would not have been forthcoming had she not been compelled to function more autonomously from the inception of treatment because of the requirements of Dr. T.'s therapeutic boundaries.

Case Three

Jill N., a 36-year-old housewife, sought psychiatric treatment soon after her husband unexpectedly announced that he wanted a divorce. Fourteen years of marriage left him "bored and unsatisfied," and despite concerns about the effects on their three children, he concluded that it would benefit each of them if they led separate lives. Mrs. N.'s initial shock quickly evolved into a profound depression. Despite chronic marital difficulties she had always anticipated "staying together through it all," and found herself "unable to imagine what it will be like without my husband." As her mood plummeted she became marginally functional and began to rely on marijuana and alcohol to "get myself up and out of bed every morning." For the first time in her life she developed suicidal ruminations, reasoning that death was preferable to "living like a shell of a woman." Her friends were greatly concerned for her welfare, but her husband became increasingly aloof and eventually left the home. Mrs. N. learned that shortly after he had acquired his own apartment a female co-worker had moved in with him. At this point she became furious, preoccupied with the thought of "running him down with his own Mercedes right in front of that bitch." She related to the therapist, Dr. W., "I can handle depression, but the reason I'm here is because I'm afraid I'll kill my husband or just hire someone to castrate him." She reported feeling so enraged that she "couldn't eat, sleep, concentrate, or even sit still," and worried about her ability to "keep functioning."

Though Mrs. N.'s fury was frightening, further discussion suggested that her threats were more wishful than realistic. She had never acted violently with her husband, even during two of his previous extramarital affairs, and she knew she would "never go to jail for maiming or killing a creep like him." She spontaneously reported that she would get "all the satisfaction I'll need by hiring a very good lawyer who'll get me a very good settlement that will make her into a very expensive whore." Reassured by her ability to intellectualize, rationalize, and sublimate, Dr. W. related that it did not seem she sought treatment because of her homicidal concerns, but because she felt emotionally overwhelmed. She replied, "I really need a place where I can talk out all these feelings." She thought psychotherapy would help her "get a hold on myself," and she added, "besides, I'm lonely for a man to talk to."

Dr. W. agreed that Mrs. N. currently required treatment, primarily to cope with her overwhelming anxiety, which he judged to be a manifestation of her considerable rage. However, he cautioned her that therapy was collaborative work that would be ineffective if she used their professional association merely as a way of avoiding her loneliness for a man. As he proceeded to explain the workings and goals of the psychotherapeutic process, Mrs. N. began to giggle. She apologized for interrupting, but said she was "amused by his little lecture about the therapeutic relationship" as she had previously been psychoanalyzed and had "heard that speech a million times before." Though taken aback by this news and his patient's behavior, Dr. W. continued to detail the limits of their relationship, stating that he wanted his views to be on record since they may vary somewhat from her previous experience. In fact, Dr. W. was beginning to set limits on his patient during this initial interview. Her history and clinical presentation revealed several histrionic traits— excessively labile affect; dramatic, overly reactive behavior; overt seductiveness; and a confused vagueness when pressed to be specific on certain issues. Though she had been psychoanalyzed, suggesting healthier ego functioning, these characteristics indicated a level of character pathology that could adversely affect the treatment. He was particularly concerned about her narcissism and potentially excessive dependency. When he finished discussing the limits of their interaction, he asked about her previous treatment.

Jill N. began analysis shortly after her marriage, when "I found myself embroiled in a torrid affair." Severe anxiety and "confusion about who I really loved" prompted her to seek treatment, which

60	*Limit Setting in Clinical Practice*

she found extremely useful in helping "discover my reasons for being unfaithful, and bringing an end to the affair." However, she was unable to remember much of what transpired during the three years of psychoanalysis. When Dr. W. asked her to elaborate on what she did recall she responded by producing the following anamnestic material.

The youngest of two sisters, Mrs. N.'s parents separated when she was eight years old and were formally divorced three years later. During an intense legal battle for custody of the children, she learned of her father's chronic infidelity, the primary reason "my mother finally threw him out." The patient's mother was awarded custody, and when the patient's sister married shortly after this, Mrs. N. became the sole child in the home. Over the next few years she witnessed her mother's romantic involvement with several men, though none of these relationships culminated in marriage. Mrs. N. then went off to college where she was "enormously popular." By the beginning of her senior year she found herself "in the extraordinary situation of being engaged to two different men." She explained that she had fallen in love with each of them for very different reasons: One was stereotypically macho; the other, sensitive and caring. Incredibly, neither knew of her relationship with the other, a situation which persisted for about a year when "I finally decided who I'd marry and just dumped the poet." Realizing that Dr. W. was somewhat stunned by her narrative, Jill N. laughed and said, "Wait till you hear the rest of it." She reported that over the years she had maintained contact with her former fiancé, periodically meeting him in another city to "spend a weekend in bed." Apart from the brief affair prior to her analysis, her former boyfriend was her only extramarital relationship, a liaison she had no intention of ending. She found him "mature, intelligent and giving . . . someone who really understands me . . . and people in general, because he's a psychiatric social worker." Dr. W. was indeed taken aback by Jill N.'s narrative. He remarked that though the acute crisis of her marriage warranted initial attention, her long-standing pattern of object relationships and chronic symptomatology (anxiety) needed to be explored. He also expressed concern about her potential for substance and alcohol abuse. Dr. W. asked his patient to think about specific goals for treatment which they could discuss during their next meeting.

Two changes were immediately obvious when Mrs. N. returned several days later. First, she was noticeably less anxious: Her affect was more contained, her speech, less pressured. More striking, however, was her extremely seductive appearance. A short skirt revealed her thighs, her bare breasts were visible through a tight-fitting top, and she was heavily made up with lipstick and rouge. The sensuality of her dress was augmented by the explicitly sexual material she discussed at the outset of the interview. Stating that sex was an extremely important part of her existence, she began to discuss her sexual likes and dislikes with her husband and long-time lover. As she became increasingly graphic in her description, Dr. W. interrupted, expressing surprise that she chose to focus on this area of her life given the concerns she related during their last meeting about her impaired daily functioning. Mrs. N.'s response was in the form of a question—she asked why Dr. W. did not want her to talk about sex. Before he could reply, she laughed and commented that her analyst had been a woman, "so there was never any sexual tension between us." When Dr. W. repeated that he had expected her to focus on more pressing issues in her life, his patient replied that she had felt "turned on" ever since their first meeting. She thought it was because Dr. W. looked like her husband, "who might be a sonofabitch, but he's always great in bed."

Jill N.'s behavior during the early minutes of this follow-up interview seemed to confirm Dr. W.'s concern about her character pathology. Her aggressively seductive style, though possibly consistent with conflict at the Oedipal level of psychosexual development, was more indicative of a histrionic or borderline personality disorder. Dr. W. based this judgment on the intensity of her erotized transference, and the rapidity with which she evolved those feelings. In light of this transference reaction, as well as her clinical history, he hypothesized that Mrs. N. characteristically defended against anxiety by sexualizing her interpersonal relationships. This patterned response necessitated clearly defined therapeutic boundaries; lacking them, Mrs. N.'s provocative behavior would serve only to detract from the psychotherapy by reenforcing her predominantly erotic interest in Dr. W., feelings that disguised underlying dependency needs. Limits were necessary to contain Mrs. N.'s anxiety at a level that permitted effective working through of the affect, as well as to protect against any antitherapeutic countertransference, since

Dr. W. recognized that he was somewhat aroused by his patient's overpowering sexuality. He shared his thinking with her, including his countertransference concerns, and proceeded to outline the therapeutic boundaries required for them to work together.

To begin with, Dr. W. insisted on a trial of minor tranquillizers. He hoped medication would facilitate psychotherapy by helping the patient feel more in control of her considerable anxiety. In addition, he was distressed by Mrs. N.'s increasing reliance on alcohol and marijuana, behavior that he felt represented a potentially dangerous attempt at self-medication given her considerable dependency. He informed her that he would insist on alcohol and/or drug rehabilitation if her clinical status suggested the need for such treatment. However, he hoped to minimize the potential for dangerous substance abuse by prescribing an effective anxiolytic agent that could be dispensed in a controlled manner.

Emphasizing the value of medical records to any treating physician, Dr. W. next requested permission to contact Mrs. N.'s psychoanalyst. He reported that he wished to discuss the content of her previous treatment, to learn which areas of her life received particular attention, as well as the process of the doctor–patient interacton.

Third, Dr. W. told his patient that he could not work with her unless she dressed differently. He indicated that her appearance so stirred his sexual feelings that it disrupted his concentration. He acknowledged that he liked to look at attractive women but felt professionally bound to limit that behavior with his patients since it interfered with his therapeutic responsibilities. In addition, he believed that as long as Mrs. N. dressed as the seductress she would continue to act out in that manner. Whether this occurred in reality or via fantasy in a highly eroticized transference, it undermined the psychotherapy. Dr. W. placed similar limitations on the material they discussed. Whereas he recognized the importance of investigating Mrs. N.'s sexual behavior—primarily because he believed it reflected pregenital, more than genital, needs—he did not want the therapy sessions to sound like monologues from an X-rated movie. That would produce the same antitherapeutic results, for the same reasons, as her overly seductive dress. He stated that he would simply interrupt the patient if he judged that she was indulging in sexual talk that was intended more to arouse the two of them then address psychic conflicts.

Finally, Dr. W. informed Mrs. N. of the *Tarasoff* decision, detailing his legal responsibilities if he considered her a genuine threat to her husband's welfare. He reiterated that he was not of that opinion; however, he had observed her affective lability and wanted her to understand the actions he would be compelled to take if he judged her anger to be only marginally controlled. He emphasized that barring that circumstance, their professional association was strictly confidential.

After detailing these therapeutic boundaries, Dr. W. asked his patient if she had any questions. She replied, "Do you think I'm attractive?" She immediately began to laugh, said she really did understand all he had said, and though she disagreed with some of his thinking she would "give things a try." However, she balked at permitting contact with her previous therapist. Believing the analyst would be disappointed by her current dilemma, Mrs. N. insisted on temporarily deferring that issue. Dr. W.'s compromise was to allow two weeks before requiring permission to speak with the patient's former analyst.

By the time of her next appointment, Mrs. N. had undergone another transformation. Far from being the seductress, she was almost demure, overtly cooperative, and responsive to her therapist's leads. This persisted for a number of weeks, affording Dr. W. the opportunity to pursue insight-oriented work relatively undisturbed by his patient's acting out. He quickly addressed the dynamic issues most responsible for her anxiety and her flirtatious behavior, the primary defense against that affect. He suggested that her parents' unsuccessful marriage, and the instability it caused throughout the family, had sensitized her to rejection and loss. She had successfully compensated for the resulting excessive dependency by sexualizing her relationships, thereby guaranteeing considerable attention from men. Dr. W. reported that via that behavior —compulsive dating in college, her dual engagement, the long-term persistence of each of those relationships, and the initial interaction with her therapist—Mrs. N. had avoided being lonely and experiencing the anxiety she associated with that condition. He believed that her relationship with each parent contributed to this defensive style and suggested that the early psychotherapeutic work focus on the feelings toward her mother and father.

At this point, Mrs. N. became increasingly seductive, and Dr. W.

reminded her of the consequences if she did not adhere to the mutually agreed upon therapeutic boundaries. He again insisted on contact with her former analyst, but she refused him the necessary permission. After demeaning and dismissing Dr. W.'s interpretations concerning her recalcitrance over the issue, she precipitously discontinued treatment. Months later, Dr. W. was contacted by a long-time colleague, Dr. K. She had called to inform him that a patient of hers, Mrs. N., had just reported that she simultaneously began treatment with both therapists immediately following her husband's departure. Further discussion revealed to Dr. W. that his colleague had been Mrs. N.'s first therapist. Dr. W. now understood why the patient had terminated treatment. In an attempt to satisfy her excessive dependency needs, Mrs. N. had recapitulated with two therapists the individual relationships she enjoyed with the two predominant men in her life. Dr. K. was perceived as the nurturing poet; Dr. W., as the sexual mate who also bore the brunt of her anger.

She had acted out a central psychodynamic issue, a situation for which Dr. W. shared some responsibility since he had failed to maintain the limit he set concerning contact with the patient's previous therapist. However, his imposition of other appropriate therapeutic boundaries eventually helped Mrs. N. to successfully proceed with one therapist and work through the emotional turmoil which had precipitated her regression. She eventually initiated divorce proceedings, though her husband was remorseful and wished to stay married, thus ending a highly ambivalent union that had brought her more sorrow than happiness over the years. Why she did not seek out another "second" therapist was not entirely clear. Dr. W. suspected that the benefits Mrs. N. reaped from her previous work with Dr. K., combined with the familiarity of that doctor–patient relationship, enabled her to continue with the former analyst, who was perceived as sufficiently nurturing and wise.

CONCLUSION

Although the preceding cases highlight the adverse effects of *specific* transference reactions, they illustrate how *all* such responses can detract from the effectiveness and safety of the psychotherapeutic process. When the usual technical maneuvers fail to contain the powerful affects of the transference, acting out behaviors can easily undermine the working alliance and/or evoke a detrimental countertransference. A psychotherapy, whether it be supportive or insight oriented, will not survive in this atmosphere, and, consequently, limit setting becomes a necessity.

Most therapists, relying on a well-developed clinical sense when assessing the need for therapeutic boundaries, impose timely and accurate interventions. However, their approach is predominantly a subjective one, based more on practical experience than objective guidelines. By focusing on the interaction of fundamental aspects of the psychotherapeutic work, this chapter has attempted to provide more definitive standards for setting limits on those acting out behaviors that derive from transference distortions. The basic principles enumerated are as follows:

First, when the patient has considerable difficulty distinguishing between the transference and the actual professional relationship with his therapist, limits are required to promote the necessary reality testing. This is most evident to the clinician treating psychotic individuals, like Mr. S. (Chapter 2), and severely characterologically impaired patients, like Lynne K. and Jill N.

Second, unchecked acting out can so undermine the working alliance that a patient becomes decreasingly responsive to confrontation, clarification, or interpretation of his maladaptive behaviors. If his behaviors render standard technical maneuvers ineffective, then further exploration of those actions may have the paradoxical effect of causing him to view the therapeutic relationship as more adversarial than collaborative. The therapist's observations and directives are ignored by a patient who has an unstated agenda for the psychotherapy and resists conforming to a less satisfying work-oriented focus. This was the case with both Jill N. and Lynne K., respectively, who used treatment to satisfy hidden erotic and dependent yearnings. The acting out may be a disruptive nuisance that merely interferes with the progress of treatment, or it may take a more dangerous form, such as Michael's threats of violence. Patients will continue to display their emotions behaviorally, which frequently serves to escalate the intensity of those affects, until appropriate therapeutic boundaries facilitate their verbal expression. Lacking such limit setting, the working alliance, and consequently the treatment, will not survive.

Third, failure to contain maladaptive behaviors precipitated by a patient's transference distortions can result in countertransference responses that merely fuel the therapeutic impasse. This is discussed in Chapter 1 and illustrated via clinical material in Chapter 5. Effective limit setting can contain negative countertransference by minimizing the aggravating behaviors that provoke the clinician's antitherapeutic response, while simultaneously providing him with an outlet for the negative feelings stirred by his patient. In effect, the therapist indirectly sets limits on himself by imposing therapeutic boundaries on the patient.

In sum, pronounced transference reactions that fail to respond to the usual treatment interventions can rapidly plunge a psychotherapy into chaos. They often initiate a common antitherapeutic vicious cycle: Transference distortions precipitate acting out behaviors that progressively undermine the working alliance and provoke harmful countertransference responses. Each of these factors continues to act upon one another, further endangering the psychotherapeutic work, until appropriate limits positively redirect the treatment. The transference feelings may promote seemingly mild acting out (such as tardiness to appointments, late payment of a bill, failure to pursue an action discussed in treatment) or more severe behaviors (such as harmful, self-directed impulsive acts). When standard techniques (for example, clarification or interpretation) help the patient understand his behaviors as resistance, the psychotherapy proceeds as a productive, collaborative endeavor. However, any behavioral expression of the transference that cannot be dealt with in this manner detracts from the treatment, and will continue to do so in the absence of effective limit setting.

REFERENCES

Breuer J, Freud S: Studies on hysteria (1893), in The Standard Edition of the Complete Psychological Works of Sigmund Freud (Vol. 2). Translated and edited by Strachey J. London, Hogarth Press, 1955
Davanloo H (ed): Short-Term Dynamic Psychotherapy. New York, Aronson, 1980

Freud S: Fragment of an analysis of a case of hysteria (1905), in The Standard Edition of the Complete Psychological Works of Sigmund Freud (Vol. 7). Translated and edited by Strachey J. London, Hogarth Press, 1955

Freud S: Remembering, repeating, and working-through (1914), in The Standard Edition of the Complete Psychological Works of Sigmund Freud (Vol. 12). Translated and edited by Strachey J. London, Hogarth Press, 1955

Freud S: Observations on transference-love (1915), in The Standard Edition of the Complete Psychological Works of Sigmund Freud (Vol. 12). Translated and edited by Strachey J. London, Hogarth Press, 1955

Freud S: From the history of an infantile neurosis (1918), in The Standard Edition of the Complete Psychological Works of Sigmund Freud (Vol. 17). Translated and edited by Strachey J. London, Hogarth Press, 1955

Freud S: Analysis terminable and interminable (1937), in The Standard Edition of the Complete Psychological Works of Sigmund Freud, (Vol. 23). Translated and edited by Strachey J. London, Hogarth Press, 1955

Greenson R: The Technique and Practice of Psychoanalysis (Vol. 1). New York, International Universities Press, 1967

Jones E: The Life and Work of Sigmund Freud. New York, Anchor Books, 1963

Little M: Counter-transference and the patient's response to it. Int J Psychoanal 32:32–40, 1951

Malan D: The Frontier of Brief Psychiatry. New York, Plenum, 1976

Meissner W, Nicholi A: The psychotherapies: individual, family and group, in The Harvard Guide to Modern Psychiatry. Edited by Nicholi A. Cambridge, Mass, Harvard University Press, 1978

Reich A: On counter-transference. Int J Psychoanal 32:25–31, 1951

Schneider I: The use of patients to act out professional conflicts. Psychiatry 26:88–94, 1963

Semrad E: A clinical formulation of the psychoses, in Teaching Psychotherapy of Psychotic Patients. Edited by Semrad E, van Buskirk D. New York, Grune and Stratton, 1969

Sifneos P: Short-Term Psychotherapy and Emotional Crisis. Cambridge, MA, Harvard University Press, 1972

Sterba R: The fate of the ego in analytic therapy. Int J Psychoanal 15:117–126, 1934

Vaillant G: Adaptation to Life. Boston, Little, Brown, 1977

Zetzel E, Meissner W: Basic Concepts of Psychoanalytic Psychiatry. New York, Basic Books, 1973

Chapter 4

Limit Setting with Inpatients

PSYCHIATRIC HOSPITALIZATION is usually indicated when an individual's behavior becomes seriously maladaptive or highly objectionable to those around him. However, placement in a treatment facility does not a priori make that behavior disappear, and its persistence within the hospital environment can readily precipitate antitherapeutic countertransference reactions that, in turn, perpetuate the patient's acting out. Therefore, the ability to effectively set limits becomes a hallmark of competent inpatient treatment. Since therapeutic boundaries must be objectively determined and reasonably administered if they are to be effective, it is essential that mental health professionals practicing in an inpatient setting be attuned to the limit setting issues specific to that treatment environment.

When formulating and revising a patient's treatment plan, the ward staff is typically aware of how the patient's hospital course is influenced by such issues as the attitude of his family, the psychopathology of other patients in the milieu, and the mental health laws of the jurisdiction in which he is hospitalized. However, the impact of these same factors on decisions concerning limit setting is often ignored, or only nominally acknowledged, which can seriously detract from the patient's overall care. Limit setting never occurs in a vacuum, especially when one is treating a hospitalized individual who interacts daily with the many staff members and patients populating a therapeutic milieu. In this chapter this point will be repeatedly underscored while specific strategies for imposing therapeutic boundaries are discussed. First, four variables are described that define the context of limit setting within a hospital environment. These are 1) the nature of the treatment setting, 2) the individual patient's treatment plan, 3) the individual patient's social network, and 4) relevant legal and social issues. Discussion of each topic explores the influence of that factor on the determination of limits, how the limits are set, and when they are effected during the course of treatment. In the latter half of the chapter the limit setting process is illustrated through case studies of patients exhibiting specific types of behaviors frequently encountered on an inpatient unit.

GENERAL PRINCIPLES

The Treatment Environment

The specific nature of an inpatient treatment environment has considerable impact on the limit setting process. Behavior that may be unacceptable on one unit, because of the nature of the patient population and the therapeutic program, may be considered undesirable but tolerable in another setting. The characteristics of a particular ward, including staffing patterns and the physical setup of the unit, also affect the way in which limit setting occurs. The central factors that define a particular treatment environment include the unit's mission, the influence of the therapeutic community model, and the effects of intrastaff process.

The Treatment Unit's Mission. Every psychiatric unit has a mission that, as defined by the hospital administration, primarily involves delivery of mental health care to a target population. Ancillary goals may include education and research. This focus, particularly the nature of the patient population, has significant ramifications in terms of the unit's admission policies, physical plant, and staffing procedures. These factors, in turn, affect the kinds of therapeutic boundaries that can be imposed on maladaptive behaviors.

Some of the most important limit setting occurs before a patient is admitted to the inpatient unit. Determining where he should be hospitalized is a crucial management issue. A unit whose mission does not include treatment of the violent patient would be improperly designed and inadequately staffed to cope with such an individual. Consequently, his admission there would create a situation in which the ward staff would be unable to effectively impose necessary limits. Similar circumstances arise with substance abusers, adolescents with conduct disorders, and patients with antisocial personalities. Unless a unit's mission is clear, and its admission policies congruent with that philosophy, the ability to impose effective therapeutic boundaries will be severely compromised.

Another aspect of limit setting related to the unit's mission and exercised at the time of admission concerns a patient's willingness to commit to specific therapeutic interventions. For example, if an acutely psychotic patient requests admission but refuses to be medicated, it would be inappropriate to admit him to a short-term, active treatment program. That hospital environment might overstimulate and disorganize the patient; referral to a longer term facility would be a more therapeutic intervention. Similarly, limits should be set concerning the admission of patients who refuse family involvement or collaboration with outpatient therapists.

The Therapeutic Community. The concepts of milieu therapy and the therapeutic community have influenced the treatment program of virtually every psychiatric unit. Although the extent and manner in which these precepts are applied vary widely, most inpatient staff accept the proposition that social processes exist among ward personnel and patients and that these processes can be used therapeutically (Stanton and Schwartz 1954; Noshpitz 1984). These interactions can have considerable impact on the limit setting process.

The original therapeutic communities were conducted according to a democratic model in which patients had equal authority with the staff in certain matters, such as passes and privileges (Jones et al.

1953; Rapoport 1960). This has been modified since questions have been raised about the appropriateness of such a model on short-term units treating patients with acute functional and organic psychotic disorders (Wilmer 1981; Islam and Turner 1982; Oldham and Russakoff 1982; Gunderson et al. 1983; Gutheil 1985). Patients in most psychiatric units retain some input into treatment decisions while the staff exercises the ultimate authority, a balance that is necessary if limit setting is to be appropriate and effective. Though patients can provide useful information about their ability to function responsibly, the final judgment on such matters rests with ward personnel for both theoretical and pragmatic reasons. The theory of limit setting dictates that effective interventions simply cannot occur without a clearly designated authority structure responsible for deciding what behaviors are unacceptable and the consequences for those actions. Moreover, the responsible individuals must have the power to readily implement the designated consequences when necessary. In a truly egalitarian community, the diffusion of authority greatly complicates these aspects of the limit setting process. The staff's authority must also be clearly defined for pragmatic reasons. On any short-term unit there are times when significant countertherapeutic and dysfunctional processes (which can seriously compromise patient management) prevail within the therapeutic community (for example, when other patients collude with an individual's denial concerning his alcohol consumption while on pass). In such instances, the welfare of the individual patient and of the other members of the therapeutic community depends on the staff's ability to intervene with appropriate limits.

Although the final responsibility for setting limits rests with the staff, the patient community can and should contribute to the process. Patients nearing discharge, for example, can socialize newer patients and educate them as to the behaviors that are not tolerated on the unit. In addition, patients can often discuss the general effects of maladaptive behaviors on the community, which is particularly helpful when an individual jeopardizes the safety of the entire community (for example, by bringing illicit drugs on the unit). In such a circumstance, confrontation from the patient's peers can be a valuable reinforcement to therapeutic boundaries imposed by the ward staff. Peer confrontation helps clarify relevant psychodynamic issues contributing to an individual's acting out, while simultaneously diffusing authority issues that could potentially be used to rationalize maladaptive behavior. There are pitfalls to this process, such as scapegoating an unpopular patient, overzealous confrontation of an acutely psychotic individual, or reinforcement of the self-deprecatory tendencies of a pathological masochist. However, enlisting the support of patients in the limit setting process is often a useful adjunct to the staff's interventions.

Within a therapeutic community there is frequently tension between rigidly consistent limit setting versus a more flexible approach. The debate concerns whether a given behavior, such as drug abuse on pass, should always be responded to in the same fashion: The answer varies with the treatment setting. Larger units, with a low staff-to-patient ratio and often a more impaired patient population, probably require a consistent policy of administrative discharge if order is to be maintained. Smaller units with highly active treatment programs have the luxury of greater flexibility. They are better equipped to tolerate some deviation from the rules without fostering increased acting out, because the rationale for such exceptions can be explained to the patient population. Smaller units can also be more closely monitored for troublesome ripple effects of acting out behaviors.

Intrastaff Process. Perhaps no clinical decisions arouse as much intrastaff conflict as those concerning limit setting. Anyone who has worked on an inpatient unit for a significant amount of time can vividly recall several patients who precipitated severe splits within the ranks of ward personnel. One group of staff members characteristically reacts to such individuals by advocating more stringent therapeutic boundaries and thus is labeled rigid and uncaring. Another part of the staff usually calls for more flexibility with the patient, earning an unjust reputation for indecisiveness. To understand why these conflicts are so common, and why they mobilize such powerful emotions in ward personnel, it is necessary to first explore the small group dynamics that frequently characterize staff interactions on an inpatient unit.

Bion (Bion 1959; Rioch 1970) described the regressive processes that occur when a group loses focus of its assigned task. He characterized these developments in terms of three basic group assumptions: fight–flight, dependency, and pairing. With each of these postures the individual group members lose the ability to function competently and collaboratively, prompting them to call for rescue from the group leader in a variety of unrealistic ways. Main (1957) and Kernberg (1975) noted that the tendency to regress to a basic assumption group is particularly strong among the staff on psychiatric units because of the regressive pull of the patients' severe pathology. Kernberg extrapolated his own concept of intrapsychic splitting to intrastaff process, deriving the phenomenon of staff splitting. He described how each of the patient's intense emotions (for example, love versus murderous rage; dependent yearnings versus the desire for autonomy) is projected onto different segments of the staff, unconsciously prompting individual members to become advocates for different halves of the ambivalence. He argued that the conflict is further fueled by patients' primitive rage, making the split even harder to resolve.

Staff splitting frequently occurs when decisions about limit setting must be made. It has several standard presentations, and the occurrence of any of the following events should raise one's concern about the presence of this antitherapeutic phenomenon. Repeated, seemingly irreconcilable dissension around an individual's treatment plan is a powerful cue. Typically, one faction views the patient as healthier and advocates negotiation to shore up the patient's failing, but predominantly competent, ego functioning. On a training unit this faction is often led by the resident physician who is treating the patient. The other group perceives the patient as hostile, demanding, and manipulative, and argues for more stringent limits. The patient's treatment plan may undergo daily revisions, or the day nursing staff may design a detailed treatment plan only to see it significantly altered by the evening shift. In such an environment, it is often difficult for individual staff members to understand that they are recipients of projections from other ward personnel.

Different patient behaviors usually precipitate corresponding paradigms of staff splitting. The split concerning a dependent patient, for example, generally concerns how much gratification to provide. The staff can battle endlessly over whether certain limits are too lax, thereby fostering regression, or too excessive for the patient to tolerate. Dependent and disorganized patients often cause an intrastaff debate as to whether the maladaptive behaviors are consciously manipulative or are motivated by organic deficits and/or unconscious impulses. Different opinions concerning the degree to which an individual can control himself are argued on the basis of these assumptions. In the case of the impulsive patient, some staff members will press for firm boundaries of tolerable behavior in order to minimize acting out, while others will criticize that course as too regressive and argue that less stringent limits will foster increased responsibility in the patient. With the noncompliant patient, some will view the resistance to treatment as a manifestation of psychopathology and define as a primary therapeutic goal the working through of emotions contributing to the behavior. Others will insist on administrative discharge.

Effectively dealing with a staff split requires that it be addressed in terms of the patient's psychopathology, as well as the intrastaff process that aggravates the conflict. The first goal is aided by such data as a detailed understanding of the patient's family dynamics. Identifying how the patient consciously and unconsciously contributes to staff dissension via distorted and inconsistent communications helps achieve the latter task. Once staff can specify the nature of a patient's ambivalence, they can reflect back that conflict as a therapeutic issue. For example, debate about whether or not to seclude a self-mutilating patient may represent that individual's ambivalence about accepting responsibility for his safety. Addressing his conflict directly often curtails the patient's acting out, as well as curtailing the contributions by various staff members which serve to heighten his ambivalence. These interventions can limit the regressive pull that accompanies splitting and enhance the patient's and staff's objectivity about the clinical situation.

It should be emphasized that contrary to popular parlance, patients do not create splits in the staff. Rather, patients' pathological behaviors and intense affects can precipitate internecine conflicts within a ward staff, eliciting neurotic and/or characterologic trends in individual staff members that ultimately promote a maladaptive group process. Therefore, when splitting occurs it is necessary to examine the patients' *and staff's* contribution to the antitherapeutic events. This involves review of the leadership and administrative structure of the unit, particularly in therapeutic communities in which diffusion of responsibility and debate about consensus decision making have occurred historically. Collaboration among staff members is obviously desirable, since increased input generally improves the quality of a treatment plan and increases the likelihood of consistently enforced limits. However, just as it is important for staff members to maintain clear authority vis-à-vis the patient community, the administrative and clinical leadership of the unit must maintain authority and be ultimately accountable for clinical and policy decisions. While allowing room for negotiation and collaboration about ward issues, the unit chief and head nurse must simultaneously maintain clear boundaries as leaders. Failure to do so may be reflected in staff splitting that is excessive in degree or amount, suggesting a posture of leadership that may be too authoritarian or, alternatively, too lax.

The Treatment Plan

The variety of psychiatric interventions now available for inpatient treatment makes differential therapeutics—the decision as to which modalities and approaches to employ in a given clinical situation—increasingly important (Frances et al. 1984). Limit setting is but one of those interventions, and the determination as to whether it is an appropriate response to a patient's dysfunctional behavior is largely based on the patient's treatment plan. This is a therapeutic contract between patient and staff that defines the goals of the hospitalization and the means by which they can be achieved. The plan is based on a thorough clinical assessment of the individual and includes the following input data: diagnosis, presenting symptoms and complaints, prevailing psychodynamics, overall level of functioning (including strengths as well as weaknesses), family situation, medical status, and history of prior treatment responses and failures. Specifically, the treatment plan must specify the *problems* that will be addressed during the hospitalization, circumscribed issues that should be stated and defined behaviorally. Corresponding *goals* should then be outlined for each designated problem. For example, a patient too depressed to care for himself may have as a goal the ability to bathe and dress unassisted. The staff then formulate *appropriate therapeutic strategies* for this particular goal. The approaches include a supportive stance (for example, accentuating the patient's strengths, while simultaneously providing structure and indicated pharmacotherapy), introspective maneuvers (for example, helping the patient identify precipitants to his depression and helplessness) and appropriate limit setting. Having defined problems, established goals, and implemented appropriate therapeutic interventions, the staff must regularly monitor the patient's progress in order to evaluate the success or shortcomings of the particular treatment plan.

Each element of the treatment plan has a general effect on the limit setting process, as well as on the specific therapeutic boundaries imposed. The problem list identified in the treatment plan guides the staff in its determination of which of the patient's behaviors should be considered unacceptable and therefore subject to limit setting. For example, behavior that might be tolerated from a chronic schizophrenic patient slated to return to foster care placement would probably be deemed unacceptable (and prompt the imposition of therapeutic boundaries) if it occurred in a hypomanic patient wishing to return to work after discharge. The different goals of hospitalization for these two patients necessitate different limit setting interventions.

Compared with an outpatient therapist, ward personnel are confronted with a greater variety of dysfunctional behaviors and work within a considerably broader therapeutic arena. Because hospitalized patients receive treatment around the clock, they are subject to limits concerning all their physical movements and interpersonal interactions. The staff must make numerous decisions affecting the patient, such as when to be more permissive than controlling or when to negotiate about certain aspects of his behavior. The problems specified in the treatment plan serve as consistent guidelines for these decisions. If the behavior has direct bearing on the issues that necessitated hospitalization and less directive interventions have failed, then limits are indicated. If, on the other hand, a patient's actions are unrelated to the identified problems and are not detrimental to other members of the therapeutic community, greater flexibility is appropriate.

While appreciating the importance of limit setting as a treatment strategy, it is crucial for both patient and staff to also recognize that it is rarely the sole therapeutic approach employed. An effective treatment plan outlines the range of interventions available to a staff attempting to help a patient achieve his goals. By indicating what a ward staff *can* do for a patient, the total plan serves as a counterweight to the specified limits that detail what the staff *will not* provide or tolerate. In this fashion, the treatment plan helps minimize a patient's exclusive view of limit setting as a punitive and depriving process.

Finally, the evaluation component of the treatment plan fosters more effective limit setting by allowing for mid-course corrections, as well as the use of different interventions at different phases in a patient's hospitalization. For example, though the staff may decide to employ confrontation and interpretation as the initial response to a patient's dysfunctional behavior, clinical improvement should prompt a progressive modification of that strategy. A recently admitted patient usually requires externally imposed, staff-monitored limits, whereas a patient nearing discharge generally benefits from boundaries that are more self-designed and self-imposed.

In sum, the relationship between the patient's treatment plan and limit setting is the quintessential two-way street. The defined problems and goals affect when and how limits will be set; the therapeutic boundaries imposed affect the patient's progress and, consequently, other approaches that may be required in the treatment.

The Patient's Social Network

A patient's social network consists of the people with whom he is closely involved and who are invested in his welfare. This usually includes family members, friends, and an outpatient therapist, but may also involve the staff of a foster home where the patient resides, his internist and/or other physicians, work colleagues, a drug or alcohol counselor, or members of a self-help group. Many writers have emphasized the impact of family involvement on a patient's hospital course (Fleck et al. 1957; Gralnick 1969; Harbin 1979). Similarly, the nature and attitudes of one's social network affect decisions about the limit setting process during hospitalization, including how the staff implements specific therapeutic boundaries.

Just as the members of a patient's support system can provide invaluable information about the patient's history and present condition, so too can they be a source of important data relevant to limit setting. In describing the specifics of a patient's dysfunctional behavior (including what improves or aggravates it), they can relate what, if any, limits the family has attempted to set and what the results have been. This can help the staff target certain maladaptive behaviors, as well as derive appropriate interventions. Contact with a patient's support system is also important to apprise those individuals about the patient's treatment plan and possibly involve them in its design; such efforts help ensure that the hospitalization addresses the major problems that adversely affect the patient's daily functioning. Moreover, since the patient will be returning to the environment of his support system after discharge, it is important that the behaviors that are required of him on the inpatient unit be congruent with the expectations of his social network outside the hospital.

When meeting with those individuals most involved with the patient, the staff should assess their attitudes toward limit setting interventions. This determination addresses two major issues. First, is there agreement between staff and family (or other relevant individuals) about what the dysfunctional behaviors are? Often a family's appropriate concern about a patient's behavior is the major stimulus for his admission to the hospital. In contrast, other families may exhibit considerable denial about the presence of significant symptoms. Second, if there is agreement about the fact that certain behaviors are undesirable, is the family allied with the use of limit setting as an approach? Though families may acknowledge the presence of frightening or debilitating psychopathology, they may feel uncomfortable with the imposition of specific limits as a therapeutic response. An assessment of the answers to these two questions will help the staff tailor the necessary limits to meet the needs of the patient *and* his support system.

Involving the family in the limit setting process usually increases the likelihood that the patient will view therapeutic boundaries as the result of concerns shared by many who are close to him, rather than as arbitrary directives of unknown ward personnel prone to abusing their power. It is therefore a felicitous situation when the family appreciates the need for therapeutic boundaries and supports the staff's efforts. This is particularly helpful at the beginning of a patient's hospitalization, when his behavior is typically most dysfunctional (and therefore most in need of limits) and his alliance to the treatment is minimal. The involvement of family in the limit setting process can foster development of the therapeutic alliance and thereby aid in the patient's acceptance of boundaries. The family also benefits from this approach by gaining experience setting limits that should be helpful in the future. The staff members act as role models and educators, demonstrating how to distinguish acceptable from unacceptable behavior and how to respond to the latter. Family members can learn to model different aspects of limit setting, such as the presentation of limits in a supportive fashion, as well as the use of confrontation and negotiation. Involving family in the limit setting process also minimizes the potential for the patient to misrepresent the staff's actions to his support network and decreases the possibility that the family will misinterpret the meaning of specific limits.

Though open communication between the ward staff and family members is in itself very important, the nature of the family's participation in setting limits must be tailored to the individual patient. For example, specific limits can be discussed in large meetings that involve all concerned parties, or in smaller meetings between patient and therapist, family and staff, or patient and foster caretakers. A paranoid patient would be more likely to respond poorly to directives emerging from a large meeting in which many people focus on his symptoms. An alcoholic individual, on the other hand, may require such a meeting to confront his excessive denial.

If the family agrees that certain behaviors are unacceptable but objects to the recommended limits for the patient, then the staff is faced with a difficult clinical situation. It must attempt to enlist the family in a collaborative approach by educating them about the need for therapeutic boundaries. It is particularly important in this circumstance to designate precisely the unacceptable behavior and the expected consequences and to closely monitor and document the patient's response to the limit setting interventions. The staff will then be better able to demonstrate to the family the appropriateness and utility of limits. The staff can also ally with the family around observation of the patient's behavior. This technique is especially useful when exceptional limit setting techniques, such as seclusion or restraints, are required. Such interventions frequently cause an escalation of the family's anxiety, which is often exacerbated if ward personnel restrict access to the patient because they observe his increasing agitation in the family's presence. At this point, the staff should educate relatives about target behaviors that represent increased agitation. The staff then designs a visit-limiting contract based on its own observations, as well as on input from the family. This approach helps limit the anxiety and feelings of loss of control experienced by relatives and can prevent a discharge against medical advice that might otherwise be precipitated by such concerns.

In addition to these educative techniques, certain families may benefit from interpretation of the dynamic issues underlying their reluctance to set limits, such as parental guilt about a child's psychopathology. Staff can facilitate ventilation of these feelings and encourage superego modification. Other families may be intimidated by a patient's psychopathology, a fear that may respond to reassurance and modeling of a firm approach.

The most problematic clinical situation occurs when family members either do not recognize that a patient's behavior is dysfunctional or are unable to accept limit setting despite the failure of other treatment approaches. Some families actively support a patient's noncompliance, for example, by encouraging him to refuse medications or to leave the hospital prematurely. This can seriously undermine efforts to impose therapeutic boundaries and may ultimately result in an untenable clinical impasse. The staff must respond to this situation by attempting to modify the family's attitude through education and appropriate interventions that address motivations for the antitherapeutic behavior. Ward personnel should emphasize the need for the family system to cope with the patient's behavior and should make clear the limitations of the staff's ability to treat the patient in the face of such noncompliance. This stance sensitizes family members to their responsibility for dealing with the patient's behavior and counters their propensity to regress and abdicate their limit setting role in the face of the staff's authority. If none of these approaches enhances compliance, transfer to another facility or administrative discharge may be required.

Legal and Social Variables

The most extreme limits that can be imposed on patients' maladaptive behaviors are involuntary medication, the use of seclusion and/or restraints, involuntary hospitalization, transfer to another institution on either a voluntary or involuntary basis, and administrative (involuntary) discharge. Each of these interventions requires the clinician to be knowledgeable about the relevant case law

(Gutheil and Appelbaum 1982) and mental health laws in his jurisdiction and to integrate that knowledge with good clinical skills and judgment in order to design and execute a workable, rational treatment plan. Sometimes this is a monumental task. The clinician, already stressed by the nature of the patient's pathology, often feels increased frustration, helplessness, and confusion when confronted with the legal and social realities influencing his management of a crisis.

Involuntary hospitalization is the prototype of a limit setting technique whose application is influenced by legal and social variables. As demonstrated by the case of Ms. E. in Chapter 1, the clinician is typically in the midst of a crisis that fosters reactivity and hampers calm and rational decision making when faced with the decision concerning involuntary hospitalization. Unfortunately, the available literature offers limited assistance to psychiatrists embroiled in this clinical situation. Much has been written about the evolution of the commitment laws (Stone 1975; Schwitzgebel and Schwitzgebel 1980; Michels 1981; Byrne 1981), but many articles demonstrate psychiatrists' inability to reliably predict dangerousness (Monahan 1981). Moreover, experienced clinicians asked to comment on individual cases note that the "right" course of action is often not obvious, and that consultations will frequently yield conflicting advice (Frances and Weinstein 1983).

Though some patients obviously meet the criteria for involuntary hospitalization, in many instances the most appropriate clinical response is far from clearcut. As a general rule, the decision concerning civil commitment should be guided by a central premise of the limit setting process: Therapeutic boundaries are employed only when less directive interventions have failed. It is therefore essential to obtain a detailed history of the results of prior encounters where the patient was, or was not, committed. It is also useful to evaluate the patient's response to alternative limit setting techniques, which may necessitate discussion with other caregiving professionals or family members. In addition to obtaining pertinent history from relatives, contact with the family can also be helpful in eliciting support during the commitment proceedings. Finally, when commitment is being considered, it is wise for the treating physician to obtain consultation from a colleague who is unencumbered by countertransference reactions to the patient.

The clinical and legal issues concerning the use of involuntary medication, seclusion, and restraint have been presented elsewhere, with both theoretical discussion and practical guidelines (Tardiff 1984; 1985). In general, such extreme limit setting techniques are used to prevent imminent harm to the patient or to others, to prevent serious disruption of the treatment environment, or to decrease stimulation that negatively affects the patient. A clinical discussion of the use of seclusion and restraint is presented in a later section concerning the impulsive patient. The issue of administrative discharge, reviewed by Gutheil and Appelbaum (1982), is discussed in a clinical context in the sections on the noncompliant patient and the impulsive patient.

The limit setting process is also affected by many social realities. Of paramount significance is the dearth of medical and support services for the treatment of the chronic mentally ill, including the unavailability of publicly supported inpatient facilities in many states. In their papers on time-limited hospitalization of borderline patients, Nurnberg and Suh (1978, 1980) advocate transfer to a state hospital if the patient is too unstable for discharge at a predetermined date. However, this strategy has become increasingly untenable in many catchment areas because of limitations on available hospital beds. Similar factors complicate the care of the homeless mentally ill. Complex sociological issues have widespread effects on the level of individual patient care, including an impact on the limit setting process.

LIMIT SETTING AND THE
MANAGEMENT OF INPATIENTS

From a discussion of the general considerations in the use of limit setting in the treatment of hospitalized patients, we now shift to a detailed view of interventions used in the management of common maladaptive behaviors exhibited by psychiatric inpatients. The case material explores impulsivity, disorganization, dependency, and noncompliance, actions that frequently precipitate admission and complicate inpatient treatment. As previously noted, limit setting is rational and effective only if it is integrated into a comprehensive treatment plan; therefore, each of the ensuing sections includes some guidelines for the general treatment of these specific behaviors. The suggestions do not exhaust all the possible clinical interventions, but rather provide a framework to guide one's limit setting approach. Also, the categories of patient behaviors should not be considered as rigidly distinct from one another. For example, how to deal with an alcoholic patient who drinks while on pass is discussed in the section on noncompliant behavior; however, because in many instances this could be an impulsive act, the principles and techniques described in the section on impulsivity might also be applied to this patient.

Impulsive Behavior

Impaired impulse control causes patients to engage in behaviors harmful to themselves (for example, self-mutilation, drug overdoses, or bulimia) as well as to others (for example, assaultive acting out). Because these actions render the therapeutic environment unsafe, effective limit setting is a core issue in the treatment. Successfully containing a patient's impulsivity requires a reasoned, stepwise approach that actively involves the individual in his own care.

First, the patient is informed that impulsive feelings are rarely abandoned in the short run and, consequently, are likely to recur during hospitalization, despite the safety, structure, and support of the inpatient environment. Next, the patient is clearly and concretely informed of the difference between impulse and action and is repeatedly reminded that any destructive behavior currently associated with impulsive feelings can be modified. Third, since dangerous behaviors are not tolerated within the therapeutic milieu, the patient must work with his therapist and the ward staff to develop strategies that disconnect the link he currently makes between impulse and action. The short-term goal of these behavioral measures is to interrupt long-standing destructive reactions to cognitive and affective cues. In the long run, they help modify the association between unconscious issues and the impulsive behavioral response. Finally, designated alternative reactions to impulsive feelings should be definitively set forth in a "safety plan," a written document that concretely defines unacceptable destructive behaviors and outlines consequences for violating mutually agreed upon therapeutic boundaries.

In this fashion, necessary limits are incorporated into the overall treatment approach. Moreover, actively involving the patient in the formulation of a safety plan enhances his sense of control and reaffirms the collaborative aspect of treatment. Patient and staff work together to identify situations that precipitate, intensify, and ameliorate the impulse. During this interaction the staff essentially lends the patient its collective ego, with characteristically healthy obsessional defenses, to help him better understand his maladaptive behavior. He begins to realize that its onset is not as mysterious or spontaneous as previously thought and recognizes that the temporal link between impulse and action can be expanded. This time lapse can then be used to pursue alternative, more productive methods of coping with previously harmful impulsivity. In this manner, the derivation and implementation of safety plans help protect the therapeutic process. Moreover, since the patient helped design these limits, he does not regard them exclusively as punishment; rather, they are experienced as predictable consequences of his decision not to employ agreed-upon alternatives to his impulsive behavior. The following case illustrates the utility of this approach.

Ms. Y., a 23-year-old secretary with major depressive illness and a borderline personality disorder, was hospitalized for self-mutilatory behavior. She had an extensive medical history, including a congenital malformation that necessitated an ileal loop ureterostomy early in life and several surgical reconstructions of the stoma. Her lengthy psychiatric history included several hospitalizations for impulsive, self-destructive acts that included drug overdoses and attempts to disrupt her abdominal stoma with various sharp instruments. Her current admission was precipitated by an upsurge of these impulses, presumably intensified after treatment of a skin infection caused by leakage around her ostomy bag.

On admission, command auditory hallucinations urged Ms. Y. to "destroy the ugly stoma." She was immediately placed on dayroom restrictions for the purpose of close observation and treated with antipsychotic medication. During the next two days she worked with the ward staff to develop a safety plan to be implemented when her impulses to self-mutilate became pronounced. The basic focus of the plan addressed Ms. Y's profound sense of loneliness, since she identified social isolation as the basic precipitant for her impulsivity. The plan, which included rewards and negative consequences contingent on her compliance, was typed as it appears below and signed as a contract between the patient and her therapist.

Safety Plan

1. If I feel unsafe I will either: (a) go to staff immediately and tell staff; (b) find people to be around and *not be alone*; or (c) ask the nurse for medication.
2. Ms. Y. is currently on Day Room restrictions and accompanied by a staff member when not in the Day Room.
3. Each shift Ms. Y. is allowed out of the Day Room without a staff member for 30 minutes, providing she can commit to her safety before each time out and tells a staff member where she will be during each period.
4. If Ms. Y. acts out self-destructively she will be placed in locked seclusion in order to insure her safety.

The staff was empathic with Ms. Y. concerning her considerable medical misfortunes and they acknowledged her understandable anger. However, rather than encouraging exploration of her intense rage staff members emphasized that the patient had choices as to how she dealt with the affect. She could continue to self-mutilate and thereby complicate her medical and psychiatric situation, or she could choose alternative ways to express her feelings that, though they might not significantly improve her situation, would not worsen it. She consistently chose the healthier alternatives, which eventually formed the basis for a more advanced safety plan that was used when she left the hospital on pass. A copy of the contract appears below.

Safety Plan for Pass

1. If I feel unsafe or under pressure I will: (a) tell someone how I feel; (b) I will try to think positively rather than negatively; (c) I will try to keep busy; (d) I will use *prn* medications; (e) I will call the hospital; or (f) I will have someone take me back to the hospital.
2. If Ms. Y. acts self-destructively on pass, she will lose all passes and privileges until she demonstrates that she can maintain her safety.
3. Two episodes of Ms. Y.'s acting self-destructively on pass will result in her transfer to a long-term hospital.

This case demonstrates the use of a written contract, or safety plan, with an impulsively self-destructive patient. However, some severely psychotic, organically demented, or character-disordered patients may be so impulse-ridden that they are unable to devise or commit to a safety plan. Seclusion, with or without restraints, may be required for these individuals in order to decrease stimulation and prevent them from harming themselves or others. Seclusion and restraints are ideally used only after the patient violates a specifically defined limit, as in Ms. Y.'s safety plan. It is therefore preferable that the staff attempt to anticipate patients' dangerous behaviors and inform potentially explosive individuals of the consequences for threatening or violent actions. Lion and Reid (1983) note that most assaultive patients have a history of assaultive behavior and give warning signs of impending aggressive outbursts. However, patients do unexpectedly lose control, and the staff should be trained and equipped to respond effectively in such emergencies. The specific procedures for restraining patients, as well as clinical and administrative guidelines for monitoring patients in seclusion, have been described in detail elsewhere (Tardiff 1984, 1985). It is emphasized here that seclusion and restraint procedures are most accurately conceptualized as part of a continuum of limit setting interventions. As such, the initiation and cessation of these therapeutic boundaries should be presented to the patient as predictable consequences of specified behaviors.

The degree of restriction imposed by seclusion can be varied according to clinical indications. Open door seclusion, the least confining, is appropriate for easily directable patients. Though these individuals are unable to tolerate the usual ward routine, they respond positively to increased structure and decreased stimulation. Patients on open door seclusion follow an "in–out" schedule that designates periods of confinement to the room, as well as times when they can roam the ward freely and interact with patients and staff. Locked door seclusion is implemented when patients are too impulsive or cognitively disorganized to adhere to an in–out schedule. The most restrictive form of seclusion, which entails physical restraint, is required for patients who pose a threat to themselves or to the staff attending them even when confined in a locked room. Progression from restraints or locked seclusion to a less restrictive situation depends on the patient's ability to adhere to designated limits. For example, a patient can be informed that one of his restraints will be removed for each four-hour period he does not make threatening statements, does not struggle with the staff assisting him in toileting, and so forth. Similarly, a patient in locked seclusion can advance to open-door status by refraining from loud yelling. During the course of each shift, the staff should review with a patient those behaviors to be modified if he desires increased privileges.

Impulsive, dangerous behavior sometimes requires that the patient be transferred to another institution or be administratively discharged from the hospital. The former course is necessary when an individual's actions cannot be safely and effectively managed on a particular unit. For example, impulsively violent patients may have to be treated within the confines of a locked psychiatric ward, a therapeutic environment with the benefits of increased staffing and a higher level of general security. The admission of such a patient to an unlocked facility may represent a failure in the screening process or reflect his precipitous, unexpected regression. Whatever the cause, recommendation for transfer must be based on clear, clinical reasons and not the punitive wishes of an angry, frightened ward staff.

A patient judged to be potentially dangerous to the community on the basis of mental illness, and who refuses placement in another institution, should be involuntarily transferred. An individual whose assaultiveness is secondary to psychosis may require such an intervention. On the other hand, a nonpsychotic patient who becomes violent on the unit should be administratively discharged, an intervention that most clearly states that such behavior cannot be tolerated in the treatment. The hospital is under no obligation to transfer this individual, since his actions are judged to be under conscious control. Moreover, transfer is contraindicated because it implies to the patient that his violent behavior will be tolerated by the receiving institution. In certain instances the police can be notified of the patient's discharge, particularly if the hospital elects to file criminal charges for any personal injury and/or property damage the patient caused. The rationale for an administrative discharge should always be carefully documented in the medical record.

Finally, certain impulsive behaviors require that specific, technical interventions be incorporated into the overall limit setting process. Management of the bulimic patient illustrates this situation. Limitations on the eating habits form the basis of a behavioral modification plan that rewards patients who refrain from bingeing or purging while simultaneously maintaining a carefully determined level of food intake. The following is an example of such a plan designed for Ms. L., whose ideal body weight was 120 pounds. It was implemented in conjunction with a list of alternative behaviors that the patient could use when she felt like impulsively bingeing.

Ms. L.'s Plan

1. Ms. L. will remain in the day room for one hour after meals.
2. Ms. L. will not use medications, such as diuretics or laxatives, that are not prescribed by her physician. Failure to abide by this will result in Ms. L. returning to Level I of her privileges.
3. Ms. L. will be weighed before breakfast on Monday, Wednesday and Friday, in a hospital gown.
4. For each week that Ms. L. does not binge or purge she may advance one level of the plan, provided that her weight does not fall below 120 pounds. If her weight falls below 120 pounds she will return to Level I and the plan will be redesigned so that she must gain weight in order to earn privileges.

Level I:
Restricted to the unit; three telephone calls a week.
Level II:
Staff-accompanied privileges; one telephone call a day.
Level III:
Family-accompanied privileges; unlimited telephone calls.
Level IV:
Unaccompanied privileges; fifteen minutes of exercise each day.
Level V:
Passes; thirty minutes of exercise each day.

In sum, the clinician designing a treatment plan for an impulsive patient should be aware of the need to integrate the necessary limits with an overall approach that helps the patient employ alternative, nondestructive means for discharging his impulses. Both the consequences for the maladaptive behavior, as well as the rewards for refraining from it, should be tailored to the nature of the patient's impulse disorder.

Disorganized Behavior

Disorganized behavior occurs when an organic or functional illness causes impaired cognition, judgment, and impulse control. This is manifest on an inpatient unit by individuals who wander off the ward because of confusion or delusional ideation, eat from other patient's trays, take items that do not belong to them, and so on. It is difficult to manage these behaviors because the impaired cognition that provokes them also compromises the patient's ability to understand, remember, and adhere to limits imposed by the staff. As a result, it is imperative that the patient's deficits be clearly delineated and carefully evaluated when formulating an appropriate treatment plan.

Disorganized patients require a particularly thorough assessment as to diagnosis, baseline functioning, and determination of psychosocial factors that precipitate and ameliorate dysfunctional behavior. Treatment plans are highly dependent on diagnostic assessment. If the etiology of the maladaptive behavior is found to be reversible, limit setting need involve only temporary measures during hospitalization. If, on the other hand, the patient is suffering from a chronic condition that permits only minimal improvement, the limits must be carefully and creatively designed so that they can be implemented by the individual's support system after discharge. With chronic patients it is also useful to carefully examine precipitants of disorganized behavior, since the most effective limit setting interventions may ultimately depend on manipulation of the external environment.

Given the patient's limited cognitive abilities, it is particularly important that limit setting be implemented consistently and rapidly. The consequences for undesirable behavior must be easily explained and simply understood. Visual cues can be helpful, such as a line of tape on the floor which the patient is instructed not to cross or a sign that serves to remind him of a particular limit. The therapeutic boundaries are part of an overall treatment plan that provides daily structure, frequent reorientation to ward routine, and regular staff contact when the patient is not acting out. If the latter is neglected, the staff primarily interacts with the patient around dysfunctional behavior; this serves to positively reenforce those actions. The staff should periodically monitor the effectiveness of their interventions, and restructure the treatment plan if the patient's maladaptive behavior persists or increases. The following vignette illustrates this approach.

Mr. B. is an 80-year-old widower who was admitted because of increasingly combative behavior at his custodial care center, as well as repeated statements that he wished to join his deceased wife in heaven. An organic work-up was essentially negative, except for residual deficits from an old right-sided cerebrovascular accident. Mr. B.'s behavior was extremely disruptive to the inpatient unit; he interrupted group therapy sessions, wandered into various rooms, stole food from other patients, and frequently attempted to leave the unit "to go home and join my wife." The staff decided that the latter two behaviors were the most frequent and significant in terms of the patient's safety and the ward routine.

The staff informed Mr. B. that grabbing food from other patients' trays was unacceptable. In an effort to prevent him from disrupting their meals, he was directed to eat at the far end of the dining table. Mr. B. responded to the intervention by loudly protesting his innocence, and raising his cane in a threatening manner. At this point he was told he would be placed in locked seclusion for 10 minutes whenever he menaced someone, a limit that was carried out twice before his threats ceased.

Mr. B.'s inclination to leave the unit in a confused state was a problematic behavior that required a more complex treatment approach. First, visual reminders were placed on the door of the unit and the door of the patient's room that read, "Mr. B. do not leave the ward." A schedule of daily activities was devised, and if the patient remained on the ward for four hours he was rewarded by a walk with a staff member. These interventions, supported by medications and the use of a brief period of seclusion whenever Mr. B. threatened someone's safety, helped diminish his wandering. However, there were still some times when he became extremely insistent on returning home. After monitoring these instances, various staff members determined that they usually occurred shortly after the patient's son had ended a visit. They asked Mr. B.'s son to contact someone several minutes before he left, so that they could begin to engage the patient in conversation or an activity before the actual departure. This proved an effective strategy that virtually extinguished the wandering behavior.

Countertransference reactions frequently complicate the treatment of disorganized patients. An initial reluctance to set limits, stemming from concerns about victimizing individuals with limited cognitive capabilities, frequently gives way to feelings of helplessness and frustration. Limit setting at this point runs the risk of being punitive and overly harsh if the patient's disorganization is rationalized as "manipulative." Each of these countertransference responses should routinely be identified and discussed when working with disorganized patients, as well as the anxiety induced by caring for individuals who are losing that which we all hold dear—the ability to think.

Dependent Behavior

Dependent behavior by inpatients is manifested by repeated demands on the ward staff. These may be overt requests for time and attention or disguised requests, such as severe regression when discharge is imminent. Because a thirst for nurturance is the primary characteristic of many such patients, it is particularly important that limit setting be conceptualized by the staff, and represented to the patient, as part of an overall treatment plan. If the staff reacts to dependent behavior merely by limiting its availability, this will undoubtedly be experienced by the patient as a punitive deprivation and can ultimately escalate his demands. If, on the other hand, limits are presented in conjunction with statements concerning what the staff can provide, the patient is more likely to accept those boundaries as therapeutic and helpful. Limits are ideally presented as part of a contract that specifies the staff's availability to the patient and indicates how the time spent with a patient is a therapeutic contact aimed at realizing a specific treatment goal. Presented in this fashion, limits are perceived less as punitive and more as a clear reflection of the reality that an individual can never have all his dependent longings satisfied. Regardless of the clinical presentation, this is usually a major goal of hospitalization with dependent individuals.

The typical treatment contract should specify exactly when the patient will meet with his individual therapist or other staff members. Questions or demands arising at other times are deferred, lest that behavior be reinforced by continually attending to it. The patient is directed to discuss his concerns during scheduled appointments, which ideally are frequent, time-limited meetings. Particularly demanding patients can be placed on a behavioral modification plan that rewards them with extra staff time if they refrain from requesting contact during unscheduled periods. This positively reinforces nondemanding behavior.

Dependent patients frequently benefit from having their therapeutic time structured by the staff. Lacking such guidance, an individual frequently uses the allocated time to emphasize his degree of impairment by describing numerous symptoms in exquisite detail. These recitations often end in requests for additional meetings in order to address other issues, a process interaction that concretely demonstrates the dependent dynamic. A useful approach is to limit discussion of certain issues, such as informing a patient with somatic preoccupations that he may use only the first five or 10 minutes of a session to discuss his physical symptoms. The therapist explains the limit by informing the patient that the goal of hospitalization is to attend to his somatic concerns and to other issues in his life. If the therapeutic work focuses only on the former, the patient will ultimately feel he has not realized the full benefit of hospitalization. The therapist then guides his patient to exploration of different issues, addressing somatic concerns only as they directly affect other treatment goals.

The discharge phase of hospitalization is particularly difficult for dependent individuals. The inpatient setting, with round-the-clock presence of staff and other patients, is inevitably more gratifying of dependent needs than any outpatient situation. Consequently, discharge planning is a crucial aspect of the treatment. The literature addresses the utility of time-limited hospitalizations (Nurnberg and Suh 1978, 1980), circumscribed periods in which the discharge date is set shortly after admission. This is a useful technique, particularly if the therapist negotiates the actual length of hospitalization with the patient. This process helps the individual develop a commitment to the discharge date as a therapeutic goal, as opposed to merely regarding it as a rejection. In addition, because the therapist enters the negotiation with a clear idea of the acceptable limits, he helps reality test the patient's perception of how long he will require the structure and support of an inpatient unit.

As originally described, the model for time-limited hospitalization advocates transfer to another facility if the patient is not ready for discharge at the specified date. Absolute adherence to this standard is not always the most therapeutic course. The discharge date can be extended *in a limited fashion* if the patient, in conjunction with the staff, can justify extending his stay by defining additional treatment goals. This is a reasonable course if the goals are deemed appropriate and if he can specify concrete markers to demonstrate readiness for discharge at the end of his extension. Lacking those parameters, transfer to another facility should proceed as originally planned.

Another concern about time-limited hospitalization is that it not be misinterpreted by the patient. If the staff focuses on the discharge date more than other therapeutic goals, the patient may view his inpatient stay exclusively as a one-sided administrative effort to get him out of the hospital. Scrupulous, daily attention to the structure and goals of the treatment plan is extremely important with the dependent patient, in that it constitutes a weaning process that ultimately enables him to leave the inpatient environment. A series of passes should be carefully planned so that the patient spends increasing amounts of time away from the hospital. If he has to make decisions concerning the structure of his outpatient routine (for example, daytime schedule, therapist, housing) then it is useful to establish a series of "mini-discharge dates," deadlines for each of the issues in question. And, throughout the hospitalization the staff help the patient determine how the dependency needs now being satisfied in the hospital will be met after discharge. In this way the patient identifies and mobilizes available social supports that he relies on increasingly as discharge approaches. The following vignette illustrates this process:

> Ms. S., a 45-year-old woman with a diagnosis of schizoaffective disorder and a history of multiple hospitalizations since age 16, was admitted because of increased agitation and intrusive behavior that could no longer be tolerated by residents and staff at her foster home. From the moment of her admission, the patient was constantly at the nursing station asking questions or seeking reassurance. On her second hospital day the nursing staff and primary therapist met with Ms. S. to design a treatment program that addressed her intrusiveness. The patient agreed that this was a primary goal of hospitalization, since it could help her control similar behavior at the foster home. She clearly required alternatives to her demanding behavior as a means of coping

with her anxiety, and consequently, the staff began to identify and devise appropriate techniques, such as listening to calming music or talking a walk. In addition, Ms. S. was informed that in order to help her use these alternatives the staff would respond to her questions and demands only at specified times. A nursing staff member met with her for 10 minutes on two separate occasions during an eight-hour shift; her primary therapist met with her at designated times three times each week for 30 minutes. Finally, Ms. S. could earn an extra 10 minutes of staff contact for each two-hour period she refrained from coming to the nursing station to request reassurance. These interventions helped the patient significantly reduce her demanding behavior within three days of admission. When the caretakers at her foster home came to the hospital they were instructed by the staff to set up a similar treatment plan with the patient. A contract was signed by Ms. S. and her caretakers that specifically outlined acceptable and unacceptable behaviors at home. Following this negotiation the patient began a series of visits to the foster home, spending increasing amounts of time there on each pass. She was discharged without incident after a three-week hospitalization.

Noncompliant Behavior

Noncompliant inpatients usually violate unit rules, ignore treatment recommendations, or pursue both of these antitherapeutic behaviors. The two types of noncompliance require somewhat different technical considerations when setting limits.

Unit rules most commonly compromised are use of illicit drugs or alcohol while hospitalized, abuse of passes and privileges, and sexual activity between patients. The unit culture usually serves as a powerful deterrent to these behaviors; however, if they arise the therapeutic community can be enlisted in curtailing their spread and controlling their effects. While the staff make clear their responsibility in enforcing the rules, patients are encouraged to exert positive peer pressure to increase compliance. This is particularly helpful when the violation involves the presence of illicit drugs on the ward, since that behavior has a clear impact on other patients.

Because limits are most effective when set in an anticipatory fashion, patients with known drug or alcohol abuse problems should be asked to sign a contract at the time of admission that addresses access to visitors and discusses consequences for drug use in the hospital and while on pass. All drug and alcohol rehabilitation programs have standardized requirements for such contracts. General psychiatric units have similar guidelines, but usually with greater flexibility that allows staff to negotiate individualized contracts with patients. Visitors are typically limited to immediate family during the initial period of hospitalization. Then, if the patient demonstrates compliance with the treatment milieu and begins to establish a therapeutic alliance, he is allowed additional visitors who must also comply with the unit regulations. Privileges are similarly advanced, and the patient is informed that a urine toxicology screen or breath analysis may be performed at any time to test for the presence of alcohol or drugs. Failure to comply with such a test is considered equivalent to a positive test result. The consequences for substance abuse while on pass or privileges should be graduated according to the seriousness of the offense, permitting the patient room for inevitable "slips" while providing reasonable limits and protecting the community as a whole. In general, a repeat offense should be treated more severely than the initial occurrence, and drug use in the hospital should be treated more severely than the same offense while on pass. Thus, an initial violation of the rules on pass may result in restricted privileges, whereas repeated offenses more readily result in administrative discharge.

Regardless of diagnosis, issues related to limit setting are frequently involved in decisions to grant privileges and passes. Obviously, concerns of safety are primary when considering increases in the level of a patient's independent functioning. If the patient is granted a pass that is inconsistent with his privilege status or differs significantly from the unit's usual style of practice, then the possibility of a staff split—and the associated errors in limit setting—should be explored. When the patient's safety is not an issue, the refusal to grant a pass may still be an appropriate therapeutic boundary if it facilitates the attainment of one's goals of the hospitalization. In this circumstance, refusal to grant a pass should be presented to the patient as a rational, therapeutic decision; lacking an appropriate rationale, the decision to deny a pass is more likely a punitive action that reflects an antitherapeutic countertransference.

> Ms. W., a 28-year-old borderline patient admitted because of
> dysfunction at work secondary to depression and suicidal ideation,
> requested a pass to go to her hairdresser. She had been in the hospital

five days and was not considered a danger to herself. One faction of the staff opposed the pass, stating that the request was frivolous and, since the patient carried a borderline diagnosis, she "needed limits." The resident treating the patient argued for the pass on the basis that Ms. W. might be displeased if it were denied, prompting her to leave the hospital against medical advice. In an attempt to resolve the conflict, the unit director asked how a pass to the hairdresser related to the goals of the patient's hospitalization. Review of Ms. W.'s treatment plan revealed that prior to admission one manifestation of her depression was the deterioration in her self-care. In light of this, her request for the pass was interpreted as an effort to better tend to herself and therefore was granted.

In many instances the ward staff must deal with abuses of passes and/or privileges obtained by patients. This type of noncompliance usually takes the form of exceeding the accepted limitations for privileges or failing to return from a pass on time. The first intervention in these circumstances is to restrict the patient, while attempting to assess the reason for his acting out. He should subsequently by informed what will be required to reacquire privileges, which usually involves demonstrating an understanding of why the infraction occurred and indicating how he would cope with a similar circumstance should it recur.

Another major form of noncompliance on inpatient units is treatment noncompliance. This includes refusal to attend unit activities, requests to leave the hospital against medical advice (AMA), refusal to comply with necessary medical treatment, and refusal to arrange appropriate follow-up. The management of such noncompliance centers on judicious limit setting coupled with an active focus on the treatment alliance. The former requires the staff to clearly delineate essential and recommended treatment goals. With regard to the latter, the staff must help the patient determine what *he* sees as appropriate goals during the hospitalization. The intersection between the patient's desires and the staff's recommendations form the basis of the treatment alliance. Outside this area of agreement, staff allow the patient to dictate some decisions while making clear that others are not negotiable. For example, the patient could be told that he must attend a certain percentage of unit activities, but can choose which one to miss. The type of medication may not be negotiable, but the dosage schedule could be.

The degree of latitude afforded the patient depends on the staff's determination of what constitutes a workable treatment situation. For example, the treatment team may decide that a moderately depressed patient who refuses antidepressant medication is likely to respond to supportive psychotherapy and the unit structure. Therefore, a decision may be made to treat the patient, at least initially, without medication. On the other hand, a psychotically disorganized patient who refuses medication is unlikely to improve without biological intervention. Since the patient cannot be involuntarily medicated unless he is an imminent danger to himself or others, the staff may decide that an administrative discharge is appropriate. Such a step is taken only after a reasonable period of hospitalization has demonstrated his inability to form a treatment alliance, after active involvement of the patient's family or support system has failed to promote compliance, and after careful assessment of his dangerousness and the reasons for his treatment refusal has been made.

A patient may be noncompliant with treatment and unable to care for himself outside the hospital, yet not be committable in many jurisdictions because he is not an imminent danger to himself or others. This places the clinician in the impossible position of viewing continued hospitalization as inappropriate and counterproductive, while recognizing that discharge could ultimately place the patient in danger. When faced with this dilemma, Gutheil and Applebaum (1982) suggest obtaining a competency evaluation for consideration of guardianship as the only workable solution to this medico-legal morass. Careful documentation of each step in the decision-making process is, of course, essential.

Leaving the hospital AMA constitutes an inpatient's ultimate declaration of noncompliance with treatment. Appropriate limits to be considered in this circumstance include a waiting period before the patient would be allowed readmission, involuntary hospitalization, and refusal on the part of the patient's therapist to continue treatment on an outpatient basis. The decision to involuntarily hospitalize is determined exclusively by the patient's clinical status; that is, whether he meets the medico-legal criteria for such an intervention within the geographic jurisdiction of the hospital. The other decisions should again be based on an assessment of what treatment approaches have a reasonable chance for success. A therapist who agrees to treat as an outpatient an individual who clearly needs the structure and support of the hospital does that individual a disservice. This usually encourages the refusal of other appropriate treatment measures, and prolongs the patient's emotional distress. In most jurisdictions, when a patient asks to leave the hospital against medical advice he is required to wait for a given period of time before being released. This period presents him with time to reconsider his decision and affords the staff time to assess the patient's current status, consider where the treatment has gone awry, and contact the patient's family. The existence of such a waiting period makes possible a problematic clinical situation in which the patient repeatedly files AMA papers but rescinds them before the waiting period relapses. Since no real treatment can occur when the patient is poised to leave the unit, the situation requires limit setting on the part of the staff. This is illustrated in the following vignette.

> Ms. D., a 30-year-old woman, was admitted to the hospital after fracturing her foot by jumping out a second story window. She denied any suicidal intent, claiming she was only trying to escape from her sister and ex-husband, who had arrived at her apartment with the intention of taking her to the hospital. They were concerned by the patient's increasing despondency which had recently included vague suicidal threats.
>
> Soon after admission, the patient filed papers to leave the hospital AMA. She rescinded the papers just before the 48-hour waiting period expired, only to file them again shortly thereafter. This sequence was repeated four times in the following week. In this particular jurisdiction, the hospital was prevented by law from involuntarily committing a patient who had signed a voluntary admission form. Because the staff was fearful that this seriously impulsive woman would leave the hospital if pressed to make a definite commitment to treatment, it failed to impose the necessary limits. As a result, her "treatment" consisted of a series of reactions to repeated AMA deadlines, as opposed to a clearly focused plan. The hospitalization had come to mirror the patient's chaotic, impulsive lifestyle.
>
> The staff finally arranged a meeting with the patient and her family for the purpose of recommending a two-week stay in the hospital; the specified goal was to help Ms. D. develop coping mechanisms designed to deal with her impulsivity and to maintain her safety. Specific pharmacologic interventions and appropriate outpatient follow-up

were discussed. In addition, the therapeutic boundary was established that if the patient was unable to commit herself to this treatment plan, and signalled that inability by again signing AMA papers, she would be discharged and the family would be advised to seek involuntary hospitalization at another institution. Although the patient initially agreed to this treatment contract, she again vacillated and signed AMA papers the next day. She was discharged to the care of her family, who took her to another institution for involuntary commitment. However, she agreed to sign in voluntarily and, because of the limit enforced at the first hospital, remained until she received a regular discharge.

As with many cases involving treatment noncompliance, the staff did not have the opportunity to see the eventual results of their interventions with Ms. D. Frequently, it is only at a later date that the noncompliant patient can accept necessary treatment, in large measure because of the limit setting that occurred during previous interactions.

Noncompliance with treatment recommendations or unit regulations often arouses an intense countertransference within the ward staff. These reactions are typically characterized by feelings of helplessness and rage and a tendency to engage in struggles for control with the patient and with one another. In such circumstances it is important for the staff to define realistic expectations with regard to the outcome of the patient's treatment. Some individuals are unable to accept appropriate treatment at certain times, and consequently, the staff must be particularly careful to evaluate themselves on the quality of treatment interventions and not the patient's outcome. With noncompliant individuals, the latter is often determined by factors far beyond the staff's control.

CONCLUSION

In sum, limit setting is frequently a crucial and complex aspect of the management of hospitalized patients. Mental health professionals practicing in the inpatient setting must be aware of both the characteristics of their treatment unit and the legal and social variables that affect limit setting. For each individual patient the specific limits must be well integrated into an overall treatment plan, and the patient's social network should be involved in the limit setting process. This chapter has outlined specific techniques for the management of impulsive, disorganized, dependent, and noncompliant behavior. For each type, guidelines were provided to aid in the precise definition of the dysfunctional behavior, the identification of specific limits, and the designation of appropriate consequences.

Compared to the limit setting task of the outpatient therapist, that of the inpatient therapist is both easier and more difficult. The hospitalized patient is, in general, more impaired and prone to more severe and dangerous acting out. However, the inpatient setting can also provide more opportunities for intervention and closer collaboration with colleagues. To maximize the utility of a hospital stay for his patients, the inpatient therapist must master the limit setting interventions most applicable to that therapeutic environment.

REFERENCES

Bion W: Experiences in Groups. New York, Basic Books, 1959
Byrne G: Conference report: refusing treatment in mental health institutions: values in conflict. Hosp Community Psychiatry 32:255–258, 1981
Fleck S, Cornelison AR, Norton N, et al: Interaction between hospital staff and families. Psychiatry 20:343–350, 1957
Frances A, Weinstein H: Dealing with the potentially violent patient who seeks help, yet refuses hospitalization. Hosp Community Psychiatry 34:679–680, 1983
Frances A, Clarkin J, Perry S: Differential Therapeutics in Psychiatry: The Art and Science of Treatment Planning. New York, Brunner-Mazel, 1984
Gralnick A: Family psychotherapy: general and specific considerations, in the Psychiatric Hospital as a Therapeutic Environment. Edited by Gralnick A. New York, Brunner-Mazel, 1969
Gunderson J, Will O, Mosher L: Principles and Practice of Milieu Therapy. New York, Aronson, 1983
Gutheil T: The therapeutic milieu: changing themes and theories. Hosp Community Psychiatry 36:1279–1285, 1985
Gutheil T, Appelbaum P: Clinical Handbook of Psychiatry and the Law. New York, McGraw-Hill, 1982
Harbin HT: A family-oriented psychiatric inpatient unit. Fam Process 18:281–291, 1979

Islam A, Turner D: The therapeutic community: a critical reappraisal. Hosp Community Psychiatry 33:651–653, 1982

Jones M, Baker A, Freeman T, et al: The Therapeutic Community: A New Treatment Method in Psychiatry. New York, Basic Books, 1953

Kernberg O: Modern hospital milieu treatment of schizophrenia, in New Dimensions in Psychiatry: A World View. Edited by Arieti S, Chrzanowski G. New York, John Wiley and Sons, 1975

Lion J, Reid W (eds): Assaults Within Psychiatric Facilities. New York, Grune and Stratton, 1983

Main T: The ailment. Br J Med Psychol 30:129–145, 1957

Michels R: The right to refuse treatment: ethical issues. Hosp Community Psychiatry 32:251–255, 1981

Monahan J: The Clinical Prediction of Violent Behavior. Washington, DC, U.S. Government Printing Office, 1981

Monahan J: The prediction of violent behavior: towards a second generation of theory and policy. Am J Psychiatry 141:10–15, 1984

Noshpitz J: Milieu therapy, in The Psychosocial Therapies (Part 2 of the Psychiatric Therapies). Edited by Karasu T. Washington, DC, American Psychiatric Association, 1984

Nurnberg H, Suh R: Time-limited treatment of borderline patients: considerations. Compr Psychiatry 19:419–431, 1978

Nurnberg H, Suh R: Limits: short term treatment of hospitalized borderline patients. Compr Psychiatry 21:70–80, 1980

Oldham J, Russakoff L: The medical–therapeutic community. Journal of Psychiatric Treatment and Evaluation 4:337–343, 1982

Rapoport R: Community as Doctor. London, Tavistock, 1960

Rioch M: The work of Wilfred Bion in groups. Psychiatry 33:56–66, 1970

Schwitzgebel, RL, Schwitzgebel RK: Law and Psychological Practice. New York, John Wiley and Sons, 1980

Stanton A, Schwartz M: The Mental Hospital: A Study of Institutional Participation in Psychiatric Illness and Treatment. New York, Basic Books, 1954

Stone A: Mental Health and the Law: A System in Transition. National Institute of Mental Health, Rockville, MD, 1975

Tardiff K (ed): The Psychiatric Uses of Seclusion and Restraint. Washington, DC, American Psychiatric Press, 1984

Tardiff K (ed): Report of the American Psychiatric Association Task Force on the Psychiatric Uses of Seclusion and Restraint. Washington, DC, American Psychiatric Association, 1985

Wilmer H: Defining and understanding the therapeutic community. Hosp Community Psychiatry 32: 95–99, 1981

Wishnie H: Inpatient therapy with borderline patients, in Borderline States in Psychiatry. Edited by Mack J. New York, Grune and Stratton, 1975

Chapter 5

Teaching
Limit Setting

The structured environment of psychiatric supervision provides the trainee with guidance, support, and, consequently, an enhanced sense of control during his early, intensive exposure to the workings of psychotherapy. The supervisory process, which allows ongoing observation of the interplay among clinical phenomena, theoretical formulation, and the effects of specific therapeutic interventions, has two general goals: 1) to help the trainee attain a comprehensive understanding of the patient as an individual human being, and 2) to provide the trainee with an opportunity to study his own contribution to the psychotherapeutic process. Each area of study has specific learning objectives.

Many have discussed supervisory goals as they pertain to understanding the individual patient (Fleming and Hamburg 1958; Debell 1963; Fleming and Benedek 1964; Schlessinger 1966). These include developing diagnostic skills (*DSM-III-R* [American Psychiatric Association 1987] classification and assessment of the level of ego functioning), fostering a general appreciation of unconscious motivations, and focusing on the specific psychodynamics of patients. These data help reveal the psychogenetic origins of a patient's pathology, his underlying affects, and the behavioral and symptomatic compromises used to forestall expression of those emotions. The trainee also studies transference phenomena, observing how the patient's interaction within the therapeutic environment mimics past and current interpersonal relationships. Finally, the supervisory process should foster a heightened sense of empathy via studied attention to individual patients and the psychotherapeutic process in general.

Those goals of supervision more exclusively focused on the trainee are primarily concerned with technical skills and countertransference issues. Learning basic psychotherapeutic technique, and expanding on that ability, requires continuous study of the impact of technical maneuvers. The student must become practiced at gathering and processing clinical data, determining the appropriate therapeutic response, and then evaluating the effect of his intervention. Attention to the countertransference toward individual patients affords the trainee a general view of his own psychological make-up, thereby heightening self-awareness. He progressively identifies the variety of behaviors that actively engage him in the treatment, as well as those that precipitate antitherapeutic reactions. He may even come to recognize a chronically ingrained countertransference that consistently interferes with his clinical efforts; however, if supervision is unsuccessful in this regard, this does not justify extending it to a quasi-therapeutic encounter. Wagner (1957) is correct when he warns that the limit for this supervisory goal is reached "if the patient as a person gets lost from sight or if the therapist tries to turn the supervision into therapy for himself" (p. 760).

Each of these general goals of psychiatric supervision addresses some issues concerned with limit setting. However, as illustrated by the first two case histories (below), the instruction is highly dependent on the clinical material under study. Educational objectives that hone the therapist's diagnostic skills can, for example, enhance his appreciation of the therapeutic boundaries required in certain clinical situations. Lacking the ability to accurately extract phenomenological data from the treatment, the trainee must rely more on chance than clinical acumen when setting limits. The following vignette, which describes the effects of intense transference distortions, illustrates the possible consequences.

Mr. L., a 43-year-old laborer, sought psychiatric treatment for the first time because "I'm sad and I have these feelings that I don't think I can handle." He began feeling "very lonely . . . especially for a woman" shortly before his first visit, but he could not identify a clear precipitant. Data from the intake interview suggested that his symptoms represented an anniversary reaction to the end of his last serious romantic involvement. The therapist, a woman, learned that Mr. L. had actually assaulted his girlfriend because he felt she was "drifting from me and not paying me any attention." She had ended the relationship and prevented Mr. L. from further contacting her via a court injunction. For months he felt "pure anger because she treated me like that," but had recently become depressed and was "worried about coping with my feelings." Mr. L. agreed with the therapist that his current emotional state seemed connected to the failed relationship. He seemed motivated to talk about his ex-girlfriend, but was vague and noncommittal when pressed to provide additional history. The therapist believed that Mr. L. was suffering from an adjustment disorder with mixed emotional features, and made an Axis II diagnosis of passive–aggressive and anti-social traits. She proposed an extended evaluation period prior to making specific treatment recommendations.

Mr. L. began the next meeting by thanking his therapist for "clearing up my head." He reported no more feelings of anger or depression and was overtly flirtatious. He praised his therapist for her intelligence and good looks, and envied her husband as "one lucky guy." Declaring his problem cured, he invited her out for a drink. The therapist's response to the extraordinary turn of events was to interpret them. She informed Mr. L. that by idealizing her he had effectively distracted himself from the painful feelings associated with his recent loss. Because of this she believed his relief would only be temporary and suggested that by working together they could help him grieve his girlfriend. Mr. L. told his therapist that he "felt normal again," but agreed to continue psychotherapy because "that means I get to see more of you." Interpreting his reply as a manifestation of continued passive–aggressive behavior, the therapist informed Mr. L. that the sole purpose of their meetings would be to discuss his positive and negative feelings towards his ex-girlfriend.

Several themes emerged during subsequent meetings. First, Mr. L. completely denigrated his former girlfriend, denying the significance of their emotional attachment. Second, his transference feelings became intensely sexualized. And, most important, he became increasingly annoyed with the therapist for not responding to his obvious advances. The treatment progressed to a point where the patient began to repeatedly state, "The only way you can really make me feel better is to have sex with me." The therapist continued to interpret his declarations as passive–aggressive acting out designed to prevent any collaborative therapeutic work, causing the patient to become increasingly angry and more demanding of her sexual attention. When Mr. L. observed that his doctor was "acting like my old girlfriend," she became frightened and requested assistance from a senior supervisor.

The consultant interviewed Mr. L. and was alarmed by the meeting. He believed the patient was developing a psychotic transference, perceiving the therapist as his former girlfriend—a particularly dangerous situation given his past history of violence. He disagreed with the working diagnosis; he believed Mr. L. had a severe paranoid personality disorder with considerable potential for psychotic regression. He emphasized that interpretation of the patient's behavior was inflammatory and not a limit setting intervention, and strongly advised the imposition of stringent therapeutic boundaries beginning with the prescription of neuroleptic medication as a fundamental condition for continued treatment. The patient reluctantly accepted the designated limits and was eventually able to grieve his former girlfriend within the now-enhanced safety of the therapeutic environment. However, his treatment had initially been complicated by an incorrect diagnostic impression that had seriously undermined the limit setting process.

Mr. L.'s case illustrates how attention to one of the basic supervisory tasks—understanding individuals as unique human beings—provides training in limit setting. A revised diagnostic assessment of the patient suggested the necessity of therapeutic boundaries, and the trainee ultimately observed the positive effects of those interventions. In this same fashion, limit setting is addressed within the general context of supervision when the material concerns another broad education goal—helping trainees study their own contribution to the psychotherapeutic process. This usually occurs when transference and countertransference phenomena are under consideration. Neophyte therapists are surprisingly unsophisticated about the existence of the transference, as well as the effects of their own feelings on the treatment. Some are almost completely oblivious to these emotions. The following case illustrates how this clinical naiveté can interfere with the imposition of appropriate limits.

Mr. R., a 20-year-old college student, was brought to the emergency room by his parents after he stabbed his younger brother in the arm with a fork. The attack occurred after "a summer of strange behaviors" and increasing seclusiveness. He frequently retreated to his bedroom, refusing entry to family members and only periodically emerging for meals. He became progressively disheveled, confused, and uncommunicative and began talking to himself, but it was not until his violent outburst that the family sought psychiatric evaluation. Mr. R. was hospitalized and, following a series of clinical interviews, was diagnosed as suffering from paranoid schizophrenia. He quickly adapted to the inpatient setting, calmed by the structure and support of the therapeutic milieu, but refused all medications because "they are inconsistent with the perfect wisdom." Wishing to avoid an early confrontation with Mr. R., his physician decided to "treat the psychosis with psychotherapy."

Mr. R. met with his therapist twice weekly for 30-minute sessions, during which time the patient was essentially silent except for periodic unintelligible mutterings or the recitation of a series of numbers and letters. He almost never answered questions directly, and in response, the therapist became progressively less active. By the end of the third week, Mr. R. and his doctor were meeting regularly essentially for the purpose of sitting in silence. Emphasizing how antithetical this process was to the collaborative work of psychotherapy, the supervisor asked why the patient had not been medicated. The therapist replied that he did not feel Mr. R.'s behavior was serious enough to warrant treatment against his will, adding that "watchful waiting" might allow the patient "to get comfortable enough to establish a working alliance." Worried by the trainee's considerable denial and rationalization, the supervisor began to explore the countertransference.

The therapist reported that though he was initially angered by Mr. R.'s withholding stance, he recently began to look forward to their meetings. He considered them "rest periods" in his day, times when he could "just sit back and let my mind wander to other things or just daydream." However, further discussion revealed another side to his feelings for the patient. Mr. R. was essentially conducting a sit-down strike—albeit an unconscious action fueled by primary process thinking—and challenging the therapist to make him talk. This became an increasingly irritating task for the trainee, who activated rationalization, reaction formation, and denial to avoid recognizing his own anger. This became clear to him when the supervisor observed that his therapeutic posture was as detrimental as the patient's silence and the family's initial indifference to Mr. R.'s withdrawal and bizarre behavior. Supervision helped end the therapist's self-deception. He recognized how he was acting out his hostility in the countertransference, in retaliation for the passive yet absolute control the patient wielded over their relationship. Discussion of more appropriate responses to Mr. R.'s intransigence taught the trainee about the therapeutic use of his feelings. He subsequently formulated and imposed appropriate therapeutic boundaries, which reestablished his control over the psychotherapy and productively ended the struggle he had been drawn into by his silent patient. This afforded him a positive avenue for expressing the competitive feelings he had previously been acting out against Mr. R., taught him the power and importance of the countertransference as a therapeutic tool, and contributed to the patient's clinical improvement.

The preceding cases accurately reflect how limit setting is usually taught within the context of psychiatric supervision. Review of this clinical data provides insight into many issues directly related to the imposition of therapeutic boundaries, such as observations about the patient's pathology, the efficacy of specific technical interventions, and the interplay between the transference and countertransference. Though this process provides the trainee with useful information about limit setting, there are definite drawbacks to this didactic approach.

First, unlike the study of individual psychopathologic conditions or pharmacologic agents, the instruction is not specifically focused. It occurs in a secondary fashion, in that learning is highly dependent on the clinical material that evolves during treatment. Limit setting warrants a more organized study of the relationship between patient and therapist, if only to inform trainees of this emotional impact each member of the treatment dyad has on the other, and should be designated as a primary educational goal.

Instruction in limit setting is also complicated by the fact that the material under study is qualitatively different from more tangible clinical data like diagnostic phenomenology. Though governed by definable fundamental principles, the process of imposing therapeutic boundaries also requires intuition and an appreciation of the subtleties and nuances that characterize an ongoing psychotherapy. Because of the subjective nature of these matters, the trainee cannot easily validate what he has been taught in the same way he might consult the literature to research a medication study or administer a battery of psychometric tests. Rather, he must place considerable trust in his mentor, a faith frequently tested by the nature of his interaction with both patient and supervisor. In fact, the greatest drawback to the current method of teaching limit setting derives from the dynamics of the supervisory process.

The impact of training on the neophyte psychiatrist is well documented (Halleck and Woods 1962; Ungerlieder 1965; Pasnau and Russell 1975). Plagued by anxiety, depression, and self-doubt, the resident must successfully cope with his emotional turmoil while simultaneously helping patients contend with similar issues. The response to such stress is varied: 1) In an attempt to offset the passivity inherent in developing psychological-mindedness, the resident may cling to the more active medical model and focus on his patients' physical ailments; 2) he may counterphobically develop rescue fantasies in a quest for omnipotence (Sharaf and Levinson 1964); or 3) he may progressively isolate himself from patients and professional colleagues. Fortunately, these adaptations are usually transient, and the basic personality structure of the resident remains constant (Pasnau and Bayley 1971) or undergoes positive change (Kogan et al. 1966). However, there are consequences of this predictable regression during training, particularly for the educative process.

In response to emotional stress, young clinicians frequently develop resistance to supervisory instruction. This has been explained as a normal phase of professional development (Sharaf and Levinson 1964), a process phenomenon endemic to this teacher–student relationship (Doehrman 1976), as well as a manifestation of personal emotional burdens, ignorance and inexperience, and relative psychological immaturity (Maltsberger and Buie 1969). Whatever the cause, the trainee frequently acts out emotional turmoil within the supervisory setting, detracting from what has been termed the "learning alliance" (Fleming and Benedek 1964) or "supervisory alliance" (Maltsberger and Buie 1969). In most instances, a healthy teaching relationship survives, producing a fundamental stability that allows the student to become increasingly receptive to observations and opinions of his mentor. However, the status of this alliance is never static; it varies in response to clinical events and the ongoing interaction among teacher, trainee, and the patient under consideration. As a result, the already complex supervisory relationship is extremely sensitive to discussion of stressful clinical issues, such as setting limits with difficult patients.

The imposition of therapeutic boundaries is usually required when disturbing emotions predominate the treatment environment. These intense affects frequently compromise the therapist's objectivity, impairing his ability to correctly assess the clinical situation and to rationally define and impose appropriate limits. Continued acting out by the patient heightens the clinician's frustration and further stresses the working alliance, as each individual experiences the antitherapeutic struggle in an increasingly personalized fashion. Though objective advice from an expert supervisor is usually welcome during such an impasse, the input may be misconstrued by a trainee whose emotions have been more intimately and idiosyncratically affected by the patient. The clinician may experience limit setting directives as criticism, prompting him to debate or reject them because of resentment and diminished self-esteem. His negative feelings can disrupt the learning alliance and ultimately aggravate the initial struggle with the patient.

The task of teaching limit setting is greatly complicated by the fact that didactic attention to this difficult aspect of psychotherapy occurs within the already stressful supervisory environment. The above issues of process and content can readily undermine the learning alliance and, consequently, interfere with instruction about therapeutic boundaries, as well as the pursuit of many other training objectives. If this is not understood by the supervisor, *all* his educational efforts will suffer; the remainder of this chapter provides teaching guidelines which guard against that occurrence. After detailing educational goals specific to limit setting, the discussion focuses on how best to present that didactic material.

EDUCATIONAL GOALS SPECIFIC TO LIMIT SETTING

If limit setting is to be designated as a primary educational objective, the trainee must first appreciate a fundamental reality of the psychotherapeutic relationship. He must be taught and repeatedly reminded that he is but one part of a treatment dyad and thus does not have a priori control of that relationship. Psychotherapy is a collaborative process in which the clinician's effectiveness is greatly influenced by his patient's ability and willingness to be cooperative. An oppositional patient can undermine the therapeutic work and also precipitate feelings in the clinician that further tax their relationship. The treatment environment cannot withstand limitless stress, a seemingly obvious fact that nevertheless must be reiterated to the young clinician who is still developing an ability to correctly assess his influence on the patient's behavior. For this reason, relating the stepwise procedure for setting limits, outlined in the first chapter of this volume, becomes a fundamental educational goal. This is a three-stage process that first requires the therapist to define and highlight to the patient any maladaptive behavior he considers to be a threat to the psychotherapy or to either of them. He then must state specifically the precise degree to which he feels treatment can withstand that behavior. Finally, he must carefully detail the consequences for the patient's continued actions.

Experienced clinicians understand this schema for limit setting as a necessary process that protects the psychotherapeutic work. Trainees frequently resist this type of negotiation with patients for reasons that range from ignorance to psychopathology. For example, many young clinicians still struggling with omnipotent rescue fantasies accept behaviors in patients far beyond what they would tolerate in any other interpersonal relationship. After identifying such an occurrence to the trainee, the accomplished supervisor should reiterate the general plan for limit setting while simultaneously trying to help the therapist understand the specific reasons for his inhibited response to the patient's acting out behavior. By addressing the process interaction between therapist and patient, this approach re-enforces the fundamental framework for imposing therapeutic boundaries and educates the trainee about appropriate technical interventions.

A second educational objective for teaching limit setting is to specifically highlight the importance of the transference relationship, since it is the major cause of acting out by each member of the therapeutic dyad. The trainee must be taught to constantly focus on the patient's transference distortions, his own countertransference, and the predominant affective interaction of the psychotherapy. Because these feelings can escalate rapidly and threaten the viability of the working alliance, the therapist must quickly identify their antitherapeutic potential and initiate actions to prevent this harmful evolution in the treatment.

A useful way to focus the trainee's attention on the importance of the relationship between the transference and the limit setting process is to highlight the *intensity* of the doctor–patient relationship. The three observations about that emotional interaction set forth in Chapter 1 are extremely useful in this regard. They are:

1. The patient can either raise hell or raise his level of self-observation, but he cannot do both simultaneously;
2. The extreme difficulty in treating someone who barely talks or listens to his therapist becomes an impossibility if that individual fails to appear for scheduled appointments; and
3. Objectivity cannot prevail in a therapeutic environment if the patient is more interested in intimidating his doctor than listening to him and the physician feels more inclined to harm his patient than treat him.

These tenets sensitize therapists to the extreme inappropriate affects caused by transference and countertransference distortions and illustrate how those emotions can transform a collaborative relationship into an adversarial one. Highlighting this interaction of feelings between each member of the therapeutic dyad and exploring how that phenomenon contributes to the success or failure of a psychotherapy may be the trainee's most important lesson concerning limit setting.

These educational goals encompass the fundamental principles of the limit setting process, its theoretical basis and practical application. First, they underscore an essential truth about psychotherapy, namely, that it is a collaborative endeavor requiring an ongoing commitment between doctor and patient to pursue the therapeutic task. Understanding of this emphasizes that when the working alliance degenerates into an adversarial interaction, limits are needed. Next, these goals illustrate and discuss specific signals that arise during the course of a psychotherapy that indicate the need for effective limits. The usual signals consist of transference and countertransference distortions and subsequent maladaptive behaviors by the patient and/or therapist. Third, they highlight the importance of a safe therapeutic environment. If treatment is to be effective, both participants must feel protected and secure while they explore the origins of the patient's emotional distress and determine appropriate remedies. Finally, by emphasizing the overriding concern for safety, these goals seek to alleviate any guilt the trainee may experience when he is obliged to set limits on a patient who is acting out. Because the supervisory setting may disrupt or be disrupted by study of the limit setting process, pursuit of these educational goals should follow specific guidelines. These are outlined in the following section.

HOW TO TEACH LIMIT SETTING

The didactic component of psychiatric training traditionally occurs within the context of two educational settings: a formalized teaching program and case supervision. This comprehensive approach includes structured and unstructured activities to provide the trainee with a body of didactic knowledge that complements his clinical skills. The formalized teaching program employs a variety of methods, such as lectures, seminars, and case conferences that usually occur in a group setting and involve a give-and-take discussion between the instructor and trainees. Newer, more diverse teaching techniques have refined these standard means of instruction. Observation of treatment via a two-way mirror provides young clinicians with an unedited view into the mysterious environment of psychotherapy. Audio- and videotaping can preserve the clinical interaction for future study and provide a comprehensive and accessible library of didactic information. All of these techniques are well suited for specific instruction about limit setting. In seminars assigned readings on relevant topics can be reviewed and related to current clinical situations. Videotapes of an ongoing therapy case can be used to study indications for the imposition of limits, the treatment issues most pertinent to the process, and the technical interventions used, as well as to evaluate the impact of specific limit setting maneuvers. A diverse library of tapes can be used to study particularly difficult clinical situations, such as the treatment of aggressive, highly manipulative, or extremely withdrawn patients.

Although there is clearly a formalized component to case supervision, the predominant aspect of this didactic process most accurately qualifies it as experiential learning. After analyzing the clinical material with his supervisor and discussing indicated therapeutic measures, the trainee effects those maneuvers and then evaluates their impact. This is basically learning by doing, but within a controlled environment. There exists considerable debate as to whether this is actually a didactic process or more a form of therapy. Ekstein and Wallerstein (1958) champion the concept of supervision as a necessary place for the trainee to develop self-awareness by studying his conflicts with the patient and supervisor. Those who adhere to this position believe the primary goal of supervision is focused attention on countertransference, in order to effect necessary psychic changes in the trainee. Tarachow (1963), on the other hand, argues that the supervisory process is exclusively instructional and never psychotherapeutic. He conceives of supervision as a predominantly didactic experience that emphasizes "the use of transference only implicitly and, if necessary, in a consciously directed manner to impart an orientation and a body of knowledge by whatever means possible, bypassing the resident's problems and certainly not bringing them to his attention" (Schlessinger 1966, p. 132).

Exclusive adherence to one of these standards influences the style of teaching, with consequent effects on the trainee. However, the debate concerning training orientation is more philosophical than real because of the most fundamental feature of supervision—namely, parallel process. Many have noted that the interaction between therapist and patient is recapitulated in the process between supervisor and student. Arlow (1963) specifically addresses the therapist's partial identification with his patient, causing the trainee to enact certain issues with the supervisor instead of objectively reporting them. Searles (1955) describes a "reflection process" in which the trainee unconsciously and nonverbally informs the supervisor about the patient's primary process by mimicking some of his pathologic behaviors. These empirical findings and the observations of others (Wagner 1957; Ekstein and Wallerstein 1958; Schlessinger 1966) were validated in Doehrman's (1976) expert study of the supervisory process, which observed the following:

[T]he therapist developed an intense relationship with his supervisor . . . this relationship had demonstrable effects upon the treatment. . . . Each supervisor was quickly pulled into a transference relationship, and certain key problems of the therapist were awakened and acted out, not only in his relationship with his supervisor but also in his relationship with his patients. (p. 71)

These conclusions are particularly germane to the teaching of limit setting.

Therapeutic boundaries required to preserve a psychotherapy are frequently necessary to protect the educative process as well. Because of the phenomenon of parallel process, trainees often recapitulate their patients' maladaptive behaviors in ways that, paradoxically, compromise didactic efforts designed to teach them how to effectively deal with such antitherapeutic acting out. This disrupts the supervisory alliance and can ultimately affect the working alliance because of the therapist's inability to objectively perceive and appropriately respond to patients' acting out behaviors. This negative impact of parallel process can occur within the context of formalized teaching and case supervision. As regards the former, a trainee may simply disagree with didactic guidance, such as indications for psychopharmacologic intervention or suggestions concerning management of a particular clinical issue. A common example involves the trainee's unconscious mimicking of a patient's defenses. For example, the predominant reaction of one therapist to a continuing case study conducted by review of videotapes was his strong disagreement with the group's diagnostic impression. His insistence that the patient was "basically healthy" prevented him from appreciating most other issues involved in the treatment. The trainee had, like the patient, invoked considerable denial, which was somewhat irrational given the available clinical data. Another example involved a clinician who challenged the worth of reviewing the literature concerned with chronically self-mutilating patients. He argued that "those people don't really want to kill themselves," and consequently, believed "there are much more important issues to discuss in this seminar." The trainee had identified with a patient's characteristic style of denigrating all attempts to help her; in a parallel fashion he espoused the futility of most therapeutic interventions with characterologically impaired individuals.

Case supervision routinely suffers from the negative impact of parallel process. A comon example concerns a trainee's lateness to supervisory hours, which frequently mimics his patient's passive–

aggressive style. Other instances of parallel behavior may be more specific, as reflected in the treatment of a professional singer whose progressive hoarseness was eventually diagnosed as psychogenic aphonia. His verbal productions, though plentiful, were delivered in a partial whisper. However, because of a countertransference that protected the patient at the expense of exploring his defensive style, the therapist brought less and less material for supervisory review, claiming his patient "just couldn't talk." In effect, the trainee had developed a parallel "aphonia" as an unconscious provocation toward his supervisor. This recapitulation of the patient's passive expression of anger affected the teaching alliance in the same fashion that transference and countertransference issues disrupted the collaborative work between patient and therapist.

Parallel process obviously has a positive side, one that benefits the trainee in the same fashion that psychotherapy fosters emotional growth in the patient. Semrad (1969) defined the psychotherapeutic process as a collaborative endeavor that helps the patient acknowledge, bear, and put into proper perspective those painful affects that adversely affect his functioning. Likewise, analysis of the parallel process helps clinicians appreciate transference and countertransference issues that interfere with accurate diagnostic assessment, appropriate use of clinical data, the implementation of required therapeutic interventions, as well as other aspects of an ongoing psychotherapy. Many of these issues are fundamental to limit setting, which is why the phenomenon of parallel process is so important when teaching the imposition of therapeutic boundaries. By recreating in supervision the stresses he must deal with in the treatment setting, the trainee sets the stage for experiential learning. The supervisor can then respond by objectively highlighting the issues contributing to the therapeutic impasse with the patient and indicate when they are being played out by the therapist in the supervisory relationship. After discussing appropriate therapeutic boundaries for the patient, the supervisor must then determine if the limits are being correctly implemented or if he must also set analogous limits on the trainee in an attempt to overcome a resistance to learning.

Though the phenomenon of parallel process is extremely conducive to teaching limit setting, it is important to remember that there are many other supervisory goals and that limit setting must always be considered within a broad clinical context. For example, when the trainee is treating a difficult borderline patient he must be taught diagnostic criteria, characteristic ego mechanisms, and appropriate psychopharmacologic treatments, as well as the powerful transference distortions and negative countertransference responses that often call for the imposition of therapeutic boundaries. This comprehensive educative approach is best accomplished if supervision is conceptualized as a complex hierarchy of learning objectives, a framework utilized by Fleming and Benedek (1964) for psychoanalytic training. They divide supervisory tasks into two types, those concerned with didactic material and those that address the student's level of self-knowledge and observing ego. The authors attend to each area depending on the needs of the trainee during the various phases of treatment. Though this offers useful guidelines for teaching limit setting, the framework emphasizes theory at the expense of practical application.

Wagner (1957) provides a more clinically relevant approach. He studied supervision from three viewpoints: method, structure, and goals. Acknowledging the difficulty of separating purpose from process, he observed that attainment of specific educational goals was influenced by the focus of the work at any given time. He proposed that different learning objectives were achieved via three distinctive teaching approaches—patient-centered, therapist-centered, and process-centered supervision. This is a particularly useful framework for studying limit setting because of its structured view of the parallel process. The case of Mr. L. illustrates how patient-centered supervision addresses limit setting. Therapist-centered supervision attends to the clinician's "blind spots and countertransference" in an attempt to foster introspection and "help him to see his influence on the therapeutic process" (Wagner 1957, p. 760). With this approach, as illustrated by Mr. R.'s case, the trainee acquires important insight regarding substantive issues (for example, his subjective analysis of clinical material) and technique (for example, how his antitherapeutic posture impeded the psychotherapy). And by analyzing the interaction among patient, therapist, and supervisor, process-centered supervision helps protect the supervisory alliance, and in turn, the working alliance.

Wagner emphasizes that supervision is a dynamic process characterized by productive and stagnant periods that reflect issues idiosyncratic to each participant. Consequently, the supervisor must carefully focus his efforts when limit setting interventions are needed to redirect a psychotherapy. If the patient's acting out behavior threatens treatment, the supervisor should discuss appropriate interventions with the therapist. When the clinician's countertransference is most responsible for a therapeutic impasse, supervision should become therapist-centered. And, if the trainee is unwilling or unable to use supervisory guidance, a process-centered approach must be implemented. The following case history details how limit setting is taught via this educational process.

Elaine B., a 27-year-old nursery school teacher, was admitted for inpatient psychiatric treatment because of delusional thinking and suicidal preoccupations. Her depression, precipitated by a surgical procedure for a correctable cause of infertility, was aggravated considerably when her father suffered a mild myocardial infarction shortly after her operation. Despite the fact that his symptoms were mild and his recovery complete, she became morbidly concerned with his welfare. She began obsessing about his state of health, calling him several times daily "to see if he was all right" and discussing his condition "with all of my friends and neighbors." Elaine B. was "paralyzed by fears to the point that I couldn't run my house or teach my students." As her symptoms worsened, she became increasingly withdrawn from family and social contacts, developed a myriad of psychophysiologic symptoms, and became convinced she was going to die "from an infection caused by my operation." Reluctantly, she acceded to her husband's insistence that she be evaluated by a psychiatrist, a consultation that resulted in hospitalization.

Mrs. B.'s psychosis resolved rapidly with treatment, but as her delusional thinking remitted, a severe retarded depression emerged. An extreme postpsychotic neurasthenia left her essentially immobilized for two months. Despite vigorous attempts to engage her in psychotherapy, and several changes in her medications, Mrs. B. remained mired in depression. She spent her days occupying the same chair in the Day Room, merely observing the daily goings-on and reading a magazine. She spoke minimally and never participated actively in ward activities. She was equally silent in individual psychotherapy sessions, which became an increasingly onerous burden for her physician. Each intervention, whether psychotherapeutic or psychopharmacologic, produced the same response from Mrs. B.—she reported that the sole reason she was depressed was because she was still in the hospital. This became an obsessional litany, a repeated judgment concerning her care. She began amending such criticism by requests for discharge, stating she would "get back to being myself once I was reestablished in my old routine." Treatment became an escalating struggle between her physician's attempts to help her confront and work through significant issues in her life and her persistent repudiation of these efforts. She began each individual meeting by requesting discharge, only to have her therapist reply that she still needed inpatient treatment for her depression. Her reaction escalated the therapeutic impasse—she stopped talking during her psychotherapy sessions. The interaction between doctor and patient had essentially deteriorated to name-calling: Each was accusing the other of being too ignorant to correctly perceive the situation, and collaborative work became impossible.

At this point, the supervisor met with Mrs. B. and was immediately struck by her negativism and overt antagonism. As she related her history, past and current, the determinants of this behavior became obvious. The central psychological issue in her life was control. She was secure and happy when she alone influenced her destiny; she felt anxious and angry when someone else held that power. This outlook on life derived primarily from her responsibilities as the oldest of seven siblings in a traditional household, and how that role affected her relationship with her father. Though she enjoyed her position as a surrogate parent, she was fearful of failing in her duties because of the criticism and punishment that such failure elicited from her father. She developed obsessional habits, such as "always checking and double-checking so that things go right for me," and consequently, she enjoyed her father's favor much more than she experienced his wrath. Though she was aware of feeling anxious in her role, Mrs. B. did not appreciate any resentment toward him for contributing to her dysphoria. She was similarly aware of her scrupulously attentive manner in her present life, and its accompanying anxiety, but was oblivious to any hostile feelings attached to that behavior.

The overriding issue of control was central to many of the circumstances affecting Mrs. B.'s recent life; her inability to deal with the conflicting feelings it aroused culminated in her depressive decompensation. The initial stressor was her infertility, a particularly painful issue as she had "always wanted a large family, like the one that I grew up in." Though she welcomed the surgery, she was disappointed that she could not "have children on my own like every other woman I know," a muted acknowledgment of a pronounced, underlying anger because she was not exclusively in control of her ability to procreate. She was also angry at her obstetrician because surgery, had yet to produce the desired results.

The second, and probably most significant, cause of Mrs. B.'s depression was her father's heart attack. Their relationship was most responsible for her predominant psychological conflict, and consequently, his potentially life-threatening illness precipitated intense, extremely ambivalent feelings in his daughter. Consciously, Mrs. B. wanted ultimate reassurance of his continued welfare, and she attempted to convince herself of his good health via obsessional ruminations. However, this pathological thinking also expressed unconscious hostility toward her father. Despite the optimistic reports of his physicians, Mrs. B. remained morbidly concerned about him. Her ruminations expressed an unconscious wish for his death, her punishment and control over the individual who punished and controlled her during much of her life.

Mrs. B.'s marital relationship also contributed to her decompensation. Issues of control, which were common in her marriage, were usually resolved in a productive fashion; the decision concerning her hospitalization was an exception. Frightened by his wife's irrationality, Mr. B. insisted on inpatient treatment, a decision she perceived as cruel, bullying, and devoid of compassion. She felt he was punishing her for being depressed, much like her father had punished her when she was irresponsible or had misbehaved.

Drawing on the content and process of his interview with Mrs. B., the supervisor offered a psychodynamic formulation of the therapeutic impasse and suggested specific limits for her obstructionistic behavior. He related this information to the trainee via a patient-centered didactic approach, concluding with the recommendation that the therapist simply stop struggling with Mrs. B. Though this sounded much easier to state than implement, he delineated several appropriate limits to the trainee, who subsequently related the proposed therapeutic boundaries to his patient.

The therapist first acknowledged to Mrs. B. his understanding that she always wanted to be in the position of controlling her fate. He clarified this issue in terms of the three areas discussed above and interpreted her persistent declarations about the uselessness of further hospitalization as an extension of that behavior acted out within the transference. He next informed her that he would no longer debate with her about the utility of continued treatment. He stated that in his professional opinion she was still significantly depressed, but that since he no longer considered her at risk to harm herself, he left the decision about continued hospitalization up to her. She could return home if she felt that would cure her depression, though her discharge would be against medical advice. She could remain if she felt additional treatment was necessary, but he would no longer tolerate ongoing complaints about the hospitalization or the silent therapy sessions, which he interpreted as her passive means of effecting control. The patient was given free rein to leave the hospital, as well as a clear statement of expectations she would have to meet if she chose to stay.

Mrs. B.'s initial response to these limits was predictable: She signed out against medical advice and returned to work the following day. Reviewing these events with his supervisor, the therapist revealed that he was relieved by the patient's departure. He felt that his increasing hostility toward Mrs. B. had probably compromised his objectivity, and although he was concerned about the patient's welfare he debated "if I am really good for her because of how she gets to me." In response, the supervisor underscored how Mrs. B. had played out negative feelings for her father in the transference, while he simultaneously explored other aspects of the countertransference. Shifting to a more therapist-centered focus, and acknowledging the trainee's awareness of his negative reaction toward the patient, he wondered if some aggressive feelings had also been projected onto the patient. The therapist disagreed with this hypothesis, arguing that his anger toward Mrs. B. was fully justified by her considerable provocation. The supervisor did not press the issue.

Several days later Mrs. B. called her former therapist requesting "suggestions" that might help her "reacclimate to life outside the hospital." She implied that the transition since discharge had not been easy. When pressed to elaborate she reported she was incapable of managing a class of 15 preschool children and was barely able to fulfill the responsibilities of running her household. The therapist commented that she still seemed to be suffering from depressive symptoms and asked what she felt she needed. Frustrated by how Mrs. B. repeatedly avoided the question, he eventually ended their conversation. The patient called several times during the following week reporting additional symptoms, but refused to commit herself to further treatment. Increasingly irritated by the patient's complaints and the sense of helplessness she stirred in him, the therapist finally told Mrs. B. not to contact him unless she desired readmission to the hospital.

During the next supervisory hour, the therapist recounted these events and spontaneously offered his feelings about "my former patient." He was relieved that he no longer had to deal with her on a daily basis and annoyed by her continued intrusion on his time. At the same time, he was "disappointed and frustrated that I couldn't win her over." When asked to consider why he felt so negative toward Mrs. B., he commented that her passively provocative style "could infuriate anyone." He felt no responsibility for the therapeutic impasse, but was self-critical for not being able to "overcome her resistance." Aware of the therapist's own resistance to exploring his countertransference, the supervisor elected to pursue the subject by focusing on the patient. Interpreting the intent of Mrs. B.'s calls as more significant than what she actually said, he suggested that she might be attempting to maintain the therapeutic relationship despite her decision to leave the hospital against medical advice. He therefore advised the therapist to call the patient and invite her to discuss her current situation during an office appointment. The therapist objected to this course, believing "it would show that we weren't really serious about the limits we set." The supervisor emphasized that he was not advocating any alteration of the defined therapeutic boundaries; on the contrary, he felt that the patient might be indirectly acknowledging her willingness to accept those limits. After considerable discussion, the therapist agreed to call Mrs. B.

During his next supervisory hour the trainee reported that his patient apparently did not want to see him because "she hasn't called back to schedule a meeting." In fact, he had contacted Mrs. B. two days previously, at which time she told him she wanted to "think things over a little." He interpreted her subsequent silence as a clear indication that she wished to permanently sever their professional relationship. Recognizing that the trainee's countertransference now threatened the learning alliance, as well as the working alliance with the patient, the supervisor shifted their work to a process-centered focus. He specifically outlined the parallel between the patient–therapist relationship and the therapist–supervisor relationship, pointing out how affects and themes in the former were being replicated in the latter. The supervisor observed that Mrs. B. was angry at the therapist for feeling controlled by him, and that she characteristically expressed that emotion passively; the delayed response to his phone call was analogous to her withholding silence in therapy sessions. He further observed that the therapist seemed angry with him. He felt that was evident during their lengthy, somewhat heated debate about scheduling an appointment for Mrs. B. after she had left the hospital. Moreover, he interpreted the therapist's delayed call to the patient as a passive–aggressive response to that suggestion, behavior again reminiscent of Mrs. B.'s method of expressing her anger. The supervisor discussed the therapist's actions exclusively as reactions to the psychotherapy under consideration, carefully avoiding any comments that might he construed as general statements about the trainee's psychological health. He concluded by directing the therapist to recontact Mrs. B. that day, and impress upon her the importance of meeting at least once to discuss her situation. If she declined the appointment or rejected inpatient treatment after that discussion, the supervisor would support the therapist's request that the patient stop calling him.

This type of process-centered supervision is required when a trainee's countertransference impedes recognition of his contribution to a disruption in the psychotherapy. Focusing on the parallel process— which emphasizes how the treatment involves a dynamic interaction among patient, therapist, and supervisor—fosters the trainee's cognitive and affective appreciation of those issues responsible for the therapeutic impasse. This approach greatly enhances his observing ego because of identification with the same dynamic forces that adversely influence the patient, making it a highly effective form of experiential learning. Moreover, a destructive countertransference sometimes requires that limits be set on the therapist. Imposing those boundaries in the context of the parallel process (that is, in the context of a specific issue the therapist shares with a specific patient arising because of a specific interaction with that individual) helps contain his resistance to necessary directives from the supervisor. The process of scheduling an appointment with Mrs. B. following her discharge illustrates the relevance of process-centered supervision to the teaching of limit setting.

Mrs. B. did agree to meet with her doctor. Appearing promptly for the appointment, she looked frightened and extremely depressed, and openly related her difficulties since discharge. She reported the resurgence of many of her presenting symptoms and requested advice as to how she could help herself. Her therapist replied that in his opinion she required inpatient treatment, but he emphasized that the decision for rehospitalization was entirely up to her since it was contingent upon adherence to his previously stated limits. Mrs. B. returned to the hospital, which provoked mixed feelings in her therapist. He was pleased she was resuming necessary treatment and that he had ultimately maintained control of the psychotherapy. However, he expected her to be sullenly withholding or openly nasty during the coming weeks, in an attempt to sabotage his efforts. Mrs. B. surprised him. She immediately got down to work, beginning with the expression of intense transference feelings. She told her therapist she felt patronized and infantilized by him, toyed with like a fish on a line. She basically communicated a hatred for him, but also demonstrated enough observing ego to realize that the depth of her feelings suggested origins beyond their two-month relationship. She soon began exploring other life circumstances that contributed to these emotions, and eventually achieved an accurate perspective on previously unacknowledged affects. Her rapid gains, which culminated in discharge within weeks of her readmission, paralleled a positive alliance she had developed with her therapist.

As Mrs. B.'s case illustrates, the need for therapeutic boundaries is most often precipitated by transference distortions; the difficulty in defining and imposing those boundaries is most often caused by countertransference reactions. This requires flexibility on the part of the supervisor, who must be able to shift the focus of study as needed. At different times during the treatment, attention must he directed toward the patient, the therapist, and the process interactions among all participants of the supervisory process. The latter focus is usually required when other educative interventions are unable to contain an antitherapeutic countertransference. In that circumstance, a parallel process evolves that requires the supervisor to set limits on the therapist in a fashion that facilitates the therapist's imposition of necessary boundaries on the patient. Not only does this help preserve the working alliance between patient and therapist, it also provides the trainee with experiential learning to complement the more cognitive instruction of a formalized teaching program. For example, analysis of the parallel process enabled Mrs. B.'s therapist to recognize how his competition with his supervisor was spurred by treating a woman he had faulted for being too competitive with him.

This chapter has also explored how similar issues endemic to the educational experience can interfere with more formalized didactic instruction concerning the imposition of therapeutic boundaries. It proposes ways to minimize those impediments, primarily by designating limit setting as a distinctive area of study for trainees. The approach, coupled with the experiential learning of supervision described above, makes the task of teaching limit setting considerably less complex and problematic. The benefits to the clinician are ultimately reflected in his more positive interactions with patients.

REFERENCES

American Psychiatric Association: Diagnostic and Statistical Manual of Mental Disorders (Third Edition-Revised). Washington, DC, American Psychiatric Association, 1987

Arlow J: The supervisory situation. J Am Psychoanal Assoc 11:576–594, 1963

DeBell D: A critical digest of the literature on psychoanalytic supervision. J Am Psychoanal Assoc 11:546–575, 1963

Doehrman M: Parallel processes in supervision and psychotherapy. Bull Menninger Clin 40:3–118, 1976

Ekstein R, Wallerstein R: The Teaching and Learning of Psychotherapy. New York, Basic Books, 1958

Fleming J, Benedek T: Supervision: a method of teaching psychoanalysis. Psychoanal Q 33:71–96, 1964

Fleming J, Hamburg D: An analysis of methods for teaching psychotherapy with description of a new approach. Arch Neurol Psychiatry 79:179–200, 1958

Halleck S, Woods S: Emotional problems of psychiatric residents. Psychiatry 25:339–346, 1962

Kogan W, Boe E, Gocka E, et al: Personality changes in psychiatric residents during training. J Psychol 62:229–240, 1966

Maltsberger J, Buie D: The work of supervision, in Teaching Psychotherapy of Psychotic Patients. Edited by Semrad E, van Buskirk D. New York, Grune and Stratton, 1969

Merklin L, Little R: Beginning psychiatry training syndrome. Am J Psychiatry 124:193–197, 1967

Pasnau R, Bayley S: Personality changes in the first year of psychiatric residency training. Am J Psychiatry 128:79–84, 1971

Pasnau R, Russell A: Psychiatric resident suicide: an analysis of five cases. Am J Psychiatry 132:402–405, 1975

Schlessinger N: Supervision of psychotherapy: a critical review of the literature. Arch Gen Psychiatry 15:129–134, 1966

Searles H: The informational value of the supervisor's emotional experiences. Psychiatry 18:135–146, 1955

Semrad E: A clinical formulation of the psychoses, in Teaching Psychotherapy of Psychotic Patients. Edited by Semrad E, van Buskirk D. New York, Grune and Stratton, 1969

Sharaf M, Levinson D: The quest for omnipotence in professional

training: the case of the psychiatric resident. Psychiatry 27:135–
149, 1964

Tarachow S: An Introduction to Psychotherapy. New York, International Universities Press, 1963

Ungerlieder J: That most difficult year. Am J Psychiatry 122:542–
545, 1965

Wagner F: Supervision of psychotherapy. Am J Psychother
11:759–769, 1957

Epilogue

WILLIAM GOLDING'S *Lord of the Flies* (1954) is a chilling description of society ungoverned by law. Stranded on an island that can support little more than a basic existence, a band of young boys struggles to survive. They soon discover that the hardships of the environment are insignificant compared to horrors they create for themselves. Though they attempt to institute ordered rule by investing a simple conch with authority—possession of the shell guarantees its holder the right to speak and be heard by all—this vestige of civilized society soon begins to disintegrate as the community progressively succumbs to its own dark impulses. Fearful of impending anarchy and possibly sensing the coming atrocities of random murder and cannibalism, some boys voice their fears and desires:

> "We're all drifting and things are going rotten. At home there was always a grown up. 'Please, sir'; 'please, miss'; and then you got an answer. How I wish!"
> "I wish my auntie was here."
> "I wish my father . . . Oh, what's the use"

Standing in the darkness, struggling unsuccessfully "to convey the majesty of adult life," the boys long for their parents. They are willing to again accept the control of grown-ups because that authority also provided them guidance and security.

Rules are irreplaceable markers of a society because they concretely define right from wrong. Whether implicit or overtly stated, benign or stringent, reasonable or illogical, rules bring order to an environment by defining acceptable standards of behavior. Members of a given group may bristle at a set of guiding tenets; however, they usually prefer them to the unpredictable consequences for actions that are neither sanctioned nor condemned. The inhabitants of Golding's menacing island voice this preference as they witness the chaos that progressively consumes their world.

Patients crave limits for the same reasons. Because limits ensure order and security, they foster the fundamental trust necessary for psychotherapeutic work. Darker impulses flourish when controls are lacking, and consequently, patients and clinicians feel unsafe if therapeutic boundaries are absent or ill defined. Though those impulses never approach the violence and horror that Golding describes—except, perhaps, in fantasy—the safety of the therapeutic environment is always diminished when patients' maladaptive behaviors continue unchecked. Acting out stresses the working alliance, interferes with the progress of treatment, and, in the extreme, threatens the welfare of both patient and therapist. It is hoped that this volume will sensitize the practitioner to such clinical situations and help him formulate and impose appropriate therapeutic boundaries in response to his patients' maladaptive behaviors.

REFERENCE

Golding W: Lord of the Flies. New York, Perigee Press, 1954